Members

Steering Committee on Future Health Scenarios

J. van Londen, *chairman*
Director-General of Health
Ministry of Welfare, Health and Cultural Affairs, Rijswijk

Dr. J.L.A. Boelen
Director of Medical Affairs
St. Antonius Hospital
Nieuwegein

Dr. E. Borst-Eilers
Deputy chairwoman of the Health Council, The Hague

Dr. H.H. Cohen
Ex-Director-General of the National Institute for Health and Environmental Hygiene
Bilthoven

W.J.C. van Gestel, *M.D.*
Chief Medical Officer
Rijswijk

Dr. L. Ginjaar
Chairman of the Health Council
The Hague

Prof. dr. J.M. Greep
Faculty of Medicine
University of Limburg
Maastricht

Mr. J.P.M. Hendriks
Chairman of the National Council for Public Health
Zoetermeer

Dr. L.B.J. Stuyt
Ex-Chairman of the Health Council
The Hague

Prof. dr. H.M. Langeveld
Ex-member of the Netherlands Scientific Council of Government Policy, Professor of Emancipation Issues, University of Rotterdam

Dr. G.M. van Etten
Head of the Staff Bureau of Health Policy Development
Ministry of Welfare, Health and Cultural Affairs
Rijswijk

R.F. Schreuder, *LL.M. Secretary*
Ministry of Welfare, Health and Cultural Affairs
Rijswijk

Scenario Commission on Future Health Care Technology

Prof. dr. H.D. Banta, *Chairman*
c/o Health Council
The Hague

Prof. dr. D.W. van Bekkum
TNO Radiobiological Institute
Rijswijk

Prof. dr. J. Blanpain
Leuven University
Leuven
Belgium

Mrs. ir. M.H. Blom-Fuhri Snethlage
Netherlands Study Centre for Technology Trends
The Hague

Mrs. drs. S. Buitendijk
Yale University
School of Medicine
New Haven
U.S.A.
(up to February 1987)

Prof. dr. H. Danielsson
Swedish Medical Research Council
Stockholm
Sweden

Prof. dr. J.C. van Es
Amersfoort
(as of February 1987)

Prof. dr. H. Galjaard
Erasmus University
Rotterdam

Ir. C. Kramer
Philips Holland
Medical Systems/Plans and Programs
Eindhoven

Dr. P.W.J. Peters
National Institute of Health and Environmental Hygiene
Bilthoven

Prof. dr. D. de Wied
Rudolph Magnus Institute for Farmacology
Utrecht

Official Observers

Mrs. dr. E. Borst-Eilers
Deputy chairwoman of the Health Council
The Hague

Dr. L. Ginjaar
Chairman of the Health Council
The Hague

Prof. dr. J.M.L. Groot
State University of Limburg
Health Economics Group
Maastricht

Dr. J.W. Hartgerink
R.F. Schreuder, LL.M.
Ministry of Welfare, Health and Cultural Affairs
Staff Bureau of Health Policy Development
Rijswijk

Dr. H.G.M. Rigter
Executive Director of the Health Council
The Hague

Dr. J. Vang
World Health Organization (EURO)
Copenhagen
Denmark

Project Staff

Prof. dr. H.D. Banta
Project Director

Dr. ir. W.T. van Beekum
Senior Researcher

Mrs. drs. A.C. Gelijns
Senior Researcher
(up to March 1987)

Drs. J. Griffioen
Researcher

Drs. P.J. Graaff
Researcher

Mrs. B. van der Lans
Secretary

Anticipating and Assessing Health Care Technology Volume 7

Scenario Commission on Future
Health Care Technology

chairman H. David Banta

senior researcher Dr. ir. W.T. van Beekum

Anticipating and Assessing Health Care Technology Volume 7

Computer Assisted Medical Imaging
The Case of Picture Archiving and Communications Systems (PACS)

A report, commissioned by the
Steering Committee on Future Health Scenarios

1988
Springer-Science+Business Media, B.V.

ISBN 978-90-481-5817-1 ISBN 978-94-017-0741-1 (eBook)
DOI 10.1007/978-94-017-0741-1

Originally published by Kluwer Academic Publishers in 1988
Softcover reprint of the hardcover 1st edition 1988

Foreword

This report, **Computer Assisted Medical Imaging: The Case of Picture Archiving and Communications Systems (PACS)**, is the seventh report from the STG Commission on Future Health Care Technology and one of a series of case studies from that project. The STG (Stuurgroep Toekomstscenario's Gezondheidszorg) was established in 1983 as an independent advisory group to the State Secretary for Welfare, Public Health, and Cultural Affairs (WVC) to assist in long-range health planning efforts. Thus far, STG commissions have examined cardiovascular disease, cancer, aging, and life styles as issues of importance to the health of the Dutch population in the future.

Obviously, health care technology is of great concern to the government. On the one hand, technology is one of the major tools to promote a healthy population. On the other hand, the costs of health care have been rising at an alarming rate in recent years. These two facts, along with the social consequences of certain technologies such as genetic screening, led the STG to establish the Commission on Future Health Care Technology in 1985. The European Office of the World Health Organization (EURO) cosponsored the project. The Health Council (Gezondheidsraad) agreed to cooperate with the project by furnishing space and intellectual and logistical support.

The goal of the Commission's work is to develop sufficient information on future technological developments in health and health care to assist planning for their consequences.

The first report, **Anticipating and Assessing Health Care Technology**, gave the overall context for activities concerning future health care technology. The government and Dutch society as a whole must move rapidly to deal with the consequences of technological change in health care. The first report provided conclusions for achieving this purpose, focusing on the need to develop a national program or system of health care technology assessment.

The second report, **Future Technological Changes**, presented detailed information on anticipated future health care technologies. In the context of STG's studies, this might be considered an 'early warning system' for health care technology.

The third report, **Developments in the Regeneration, Repair and Reorganization of Nervous Tissue**, focused on future applications of neurosciences, especially regarding Alzheimer's disease, Parkinson's disease, and accidents involving nervous system trauma.

The fourth report, **Health Care Applications of Lasers: The Future Treatment of Coronary Artery Disease**, presents a general introduction to lasers in health care, although more detailed information is presented in Volume II. The main purpose of this case study is to examine the possible impacts of one application of lasers: the treatment of coronary artery disease.

The fifth report, **Developments in Genetic Testing**, examines another application of the new biotechnology, the rapidly developing field of genetics. The genetic revolution has now truly begun and it will transform the ways that society deals with its genetic inheritance. The implications of this new technology are far-reaching. The report explores some of these implications and suggests the importance of careful monitoring of this field.

The sixth report, **Applications of the New Biotechnology: The Case of Vaccines**, discusses developments in the new biotechnology. The ability to directly manipulate the genetic structure of organisms has lead to dramatic changes in biological research, and is now beginning to transform practical technology as well. The report presents some of the new developments in diagnostic and therapeutic technologies. The main purpose of the report, however, is to point out the potential applications in vaccine development and possible future impacts of this field on the health of the Netherlands population.

This report, **Computer Assisted Medical Imaging: The Case of Picture Archiving and Communications Systems (PACS)**, presents information on an important new technology. Since the early 1970s, departments of radiology have gradually turned to imaging with computers, and there are now predictions that all medical images, including conventional x-rays, will be computerized. Such a move would have great potential advantages, but the costs to the health care system and society would also be large. It is important for Dutch society to become aware of these developments and to determine the best course of future action.

The final report from the project on future health care technology, **Potentials for Home Care Technology**, gives an overview of present and future developments in an important and often-neglected field of health care. The report also describes and analyses the home care system of the Netherlands, and conlcudes that the home care system is not structured to be receptive to technology. Therefore, the report suggests ways that the home care system could be improved.

As Chairman of the STG, I am delighted to present this report, and I thank the Commission very sincerely for its rapid and excellent work. The government expects to see changes in policies toward health care technology, and I am certain that the report will be a substantial help in that process of change.

The report was prepared by the Commission's staff, which is listed in this report. The staff was led by Dr. David Banta, an American who agreed to spend two years with the STG chairing the Commission. The decision to invite Dr. Banta to the Netherlands was a recognition of the international nature of issues concerning health care technology. I would also like to point out the presence of a Swede, Dr. Henry Danielson, and a Belgian, Professor Jan Blanpain, on the Commission. Dr. Johannes Vang from WHO/EURO was an official observer on the Commission. We are particularly grateful to these outside guests.

The reports have been developed with the help of experts and reviewed by the Commission and by many other individuals and groups representing a wide range of disciplines and perspectives. We are grateful for their many contributions. As with all STG reports, however, the content of the report is the responsibility of the Commission and the STG and does not necessarily represent the position of any of those who assisted or of the Ministry of WVC.

J. van Londen
Chairman, STG

Preface

As noted in the Foreword, this report is one of several volumes resulting from this study of future health care technology.

The purpose of the study, as formulated by the STG, was to analyze future health care technology. Part of the task was to develop an 'early warning system' for health care technology. The primary goal of the project was to develop a list or description of a number of possible and probable future health care technologies, as well as information on their importance. Within the limits of time and money, this has been done. However, given the vast number of possible future health care technologies, complete information on the importance of each area could not be developed in any depth for all technology.

Therefore, four specific technologies were chosen and were prospectively assessed. These future technologies were examined in more depth, looking particularly at their future health and policy implications. Subsequently, the project was extended to September 1986, and two additional technologies were chosen for assessment.

The total anticipated output of the project is as follows:

Volume 1. GENERAL CONSIDERATIONS AND POLICY RECOMMENDATIONS

Volume 2. FUTURE TECHNOLOGICAL CHANGES

Volume 3. DEVELOPMENTS IN THE REGENERATION, REPAIR AND REORGANIZATION OF NERVOUS TISSUE

Volume 4. HEALTH CARE APPLICATIONS OF LASERS: THE FUTURE TREATMENT OF CORONARY ARTERY DISEASE

Volume 5. DEVELOPMENTS IN GENETIC TESTING

Volume 6. APPLICATIONS OF THE NEW BIOTECHNOLOGY: THE CASE OF VACCINES

Volume 7. COMPUTER-ASSISTED MEDICAL IMAGING: The Case of Picture Archiving and Communications Systems (PACS)

Volume 8. POTENTIALS FOR HOME CARE TECHNOLOGY

The first report was addressed to an important purpose. The Commission reached the tentative conclusion early in its deliberations that a system for identifying future health care technology would be of limited benefit on its own. The Netherlands does not have an organized system for technology assessment in health care, and therefore information on the benefits, risks, financial costs, and social implications of technology is not available for new or established technology, generally speaking. The Commission saw the need for such a system. Studies aimed at the identification and assessment of future health care technologies must be developed within such a context, the Commission concluded. Therefore, Volume I was developed as an overall policy document, and contains summary material on future technologies. This report gives the detailed information on the same technologies and technological areas.

The second report presented overall information on future health care technology. The report was based on information obtained from surveys done in the United States and in Europe.

The case studies are intended to examine important areas of future (and emerging) health care technology. However, many other potential subjects and applications could be examined. This case study, then, is only an example of what may be possible in evaluating the impacts of future health care technology.

Technological developments in health care are occurring rapidly, and the information on future technologies in these report will rapidly become out-of-date. The Commission is aware of this fact, and hopes that it will be possible to continue an 'early warning system' that will periodically update such information and assess specific technologies.

The Ministry of Economical Affairs (EZ) supported the development of this case study because of the potential for industrial development in computer assisted medical imaging. Therefore, one of the questions in this study is how to encourage industry to become more active in this area. Dr.ir. van Beekum was therefore assigned to this part of the project.

This report is primarily addressed to policy makers and to those who are interested in national level policy making. At the same time, the Commission believes that the information in this report is an important basis for future activities in health care technology assessment in Netherlands and in other countries.

Dr. H. David Banta
Chairman
Commission on Future Health Care Technology

and

Dr. ir. W.T. van Beekum
Senior Researcher

Table of Contents

Introduction

The field of medical imaging - the use of images of the inside of the human body for the purpose of medical diagnosis - began with the discovery of x-rays in 1895. The x-ray image is now a pervasive and familiar part of health care services. Although technological improvements have occurred and new methods of imaging were incorporated into departments of radiology during the past decades, the basic structure of these services was set by early in the 20th century.

A quiet revolution began, however, in 1972, with the introduction of the computed tomography (CT) scanner (7,60). The CT scanner was an early clinical application of computers, which were not practical until the 1950s and 1960s. It uses digital (numeric) data for the first time to construct images of the inside of the human body.

Medical imaging is already one of the most important parts of the health care system. It is hardly conceivable now that a surgical procedure would be done without an x-ray or other image to guide the surgeon. Treatment of conditions from bone fractures to pneumonia depend on such images. The technology of the x-ray has affected the structure of health care services; the department of radiology is usually centrally sited in the hospital and the medical specialists who provide these services and interpret the images, radiologists, are valued and prestigious members of the medical profession. At the same time, this area of health care is one of the most visible and most regulated. X-rays are a form of ionizing radiation, so cause mutagenic processes that can lead to cancer and other serious health problems. The services also are not cheap, making up perhaps 3 to 5 percent of the national health expenditure in industrialized countries. The placement of such high capital devices as CT scanners is regulated by the governments of most industrialized countries.

As medical imaging continues to develop - and as the computer becomes more and more central to the field - a variety of policy issues will become visible. The main one facing a country such as the Netherlands is, should the large capital investments required for computer-based imaging systems of the future be made? A subsidiary question concerns the type of evaluation and monitoring strategy needed to help future decision-making.

This report presents basic descriptive information on computer assisted medical imaging. It emphasizes the growing use of digital or numeric data in this field, and the role of the computer now and in the future. Computer assisted medical imaging is already a rapidly growing field.

The basic decision concerns how to organize these services. Should systems totally based on computers be encouraged? Such systems are known as **Picture Archiving and Communications Systems (PACS)** (74). A PACS uses the computer not only to collect the data and to analyze it to reconstruct an image, but to move it from place to place (**communication**) and to store and retrieve it (**archiving**). Thus, it seems certain that computer assisted medical imaging will continue to grow. The question concerns efficient handling of the data obtained from such imaging systems.

The emphasis in this report is on developments in computer assisted medical imaging. This requires a change in perspective for the reader. The natural tendency is to compare computer assisted imaging with the previous film systems. This is probably analagous to the reports of predictions of the future importance of telephones done early in this century based on the number of letters that people wrote! Although ultimate developments and applications in computer assisted medical imaging cannot be predicted in detail, it does seem clear that eventually dramatic change will result (19). For example, it seems likely that imaging work stations will proliferate both inside and outside the institution and physician's office, increasing the use of diagnostic imaging (17). The technology could bring the radiologist and referring physician in closer communication to improve the diagnostic process.

The diagnostic process is already changing in significant ways. The proliferation of diagnostic tests and techniques has led, in some instances, to technical teams who respond to clinician requests, and one of whose tasks is to integrate diagnostic information. In time, a further development could be a highly automated diagnostic process. Systems dependent on computers for interpretation of images could also become widespread (31).

The **organization** of the report is as follows: The first section provides an overview of past, present, and future developments, including industrial involvements. The second section discusses the health care implications of such developments. The third section examines benefits and costs of computer-assisted imaging, focusing on financial issues. The fourth section discusses international aspects of the field. And the fifth section presents conclusions for health care policy, for industry, and for research.

Section 1 – Background on Computer Assisted Medical Imaging

Diagnosis is a critical part of health care. Diagnosis is the process of determining a patient's illness from his or her complaints and from other sources of information. Most people go to physicians because of symptoms; it is then the role of the physician or other health care provider to find an explanation for those symptoms. Imaging is different in some respects from other diagnostic tools, since the location and size of a lesion can be determined, and sometimes its stage of development as well. In addition, the diagnosis determine the course of medical intervention, including the possibility of cure. Images are also often used in follow-up of therapy to determines its effectiveness. In addition, imaging is sometimes used in screening programs to identify early disease that has not yet caused symptoms.

The devices that produce medical images provide valuable diagnostic information; in many cases, this information can be critical for medical decisions. The making of images or pictures of the inside of the human body is a relatively recent activity in medicine, but it has in itself transformed medical diagnosis and treatment. The development of computer assisted medical imaging has led to further dramatic changes, still underway. This Section describes these changes, and discusses probable future developments.

Historical Background

In 1895, Wilhelm Roentgen, a Professor of Physics in Wuerzburg, Bavaria, noticed, while carrying out experiments with a cathode ray tube, that a fluorescent screen lying about a meter away began to glow. This observation led to the discovery of x-rays. Roentgen quickly discovered that the new radiation could penetrate solid objects. He noted that they did not so easily pass dense substances, such as bone. "If the hand be held before the fluorescent screen," wrote Roentgen, "the shadow shows the bones darkly with only faint outlines of the surrounding tissues" (64, p. 58-59). Roentgen found that the images could be captured on photographic plates as well as on fluorescent screens. This was the beginning of medical imaging.

The x-ray device was rapidly accepted by the medical profession. Within weeks of the discovery, medical journals in the United States and Great Britain printed articles describing shadow pictures of arm bones, leg bones, and gall and kidney stones (64, p. 62). The advantages with bone fractures and foreign objects in the body were quickly seen. By 1899, x-rays were being used to diagnose diseases of the lungs, and bismuth was used beginning in 1896 to make pictures of the gastrointestinal tract from end to end. X-ray machines were on the market by 1896 at a cost of about US$50, and shortly afterwards, the fluoroscope appeared. It was an x-ray generating apparatus with a screen coated with fluorescent material (64, p. 62). The fluoroscope allowed an instant view of the body and could show organs and tissues in motion.

The early decades of the 20th century saw the institutionalization of x-ray. Departments of radiology were established in the early decades of the century, and they expanded rapidly in the 1920s (70, p. 46). A specialized group of physicians, called radiologists, gradually formed to oversee the process of taking x-ray images and to provide expert interpretation of them. During the 1920s and 1930s, many departments of radiology were directed by non-physicians (69, p. 226;70, p. 46). The medical specialty was formally established in the 1930s (69, p. 325;70, 1966, p. 46-47).

The x-ray produced significant changes in the methods physicians used to diagnose illness. Previously, the physician mostly worked alone, gathering diagnostic information directly from the patient. With x-rays, several physicians could look at an x-ray image together simultaneously, leading to discussion and group diagnosis. In addition, the patient did not need to be present while the x-ray was examined and discussed (64, p. 68).

Although there were continual improvements in x-ray technology during the decades leading up to 1970, the basic technology had been developed before 1900. The major change in conventional x-ray has been to reduce the radiation dose given to patients during the procedure (27). Since x-rays are known to be associated health problems, it can be assumed that this change is of benefit to patients. In the period following World War II, new imaging modalities such as nuclear medicine and ultrasound found increasing use, but produced no striking changes in methods of diagnosis. The next dramatic change in medical imaging came with the development of the CT scanner, which was in fact the introduction of computer assisted medical imaging. The mathematical theory that allowed the CT scanner was put forward by Radon in 1917 (8). However, technological advances such as the development of computers were necessary before this theory could be applied practically. The first workable CT device was built in 1963. The EMI company in Britain produced the first commercial device. The prototype was tested in 1971 and EMI began marketing the CT scanner in 1972 (8).

The **computed tomography (CT) scanner** is a diagnostic device that combines x-ray equipment with a computer and a display monitor to produce images of cross sections of the human body (60; 61). The earliest x-ray films (and conventional x-ray films today) depended on the exposure of film to x-rays to measure the amount of radiation that passes through different parts of the body. The CT scanner passes x-rays through the body from a number of different points, measures the amount of radiation passing through the body, and uses the data to mathematically reconstruct the image or picture. The advantages of this form of imaging are that a picture can be constructed (different from the shadows seen on x-ray) and that organs that are ordinarily super-imposed on x-rays can be seen separately. In addition, CT scanning makes the reconstruction of three-dimensional images possible. The data are in digital (computer-readable numbers) form, leading to the terms 'digital imaging' and 'digitization.' This means that the information from the x-ray (or other energy source in other methods) passing through the body is converted to electronic codes representing numbers in the computer and used to produce or reconstruct an image that is then presented on a display monitor. The data can be stored in the computer, disk, or other medium, or the image can be photographed and stored in that form.

The diffusion of the CT scanner may have been the fastest of any health care technology in history (8). It was greeted by the medical profession with great enthusiasm. Although the price was high, about US$250,000, companies scrambled to enter the market and initial profits were high. In the United States, the first CT scanner was installed in 1973. In the Netherlands, the first scanner was installed in 1975. The United States now has about 2,000 CT scanners, for a population rate of over 10 per million. The Netherlands has 45 CT scanners, about 3 for every million people.

Digitization of data from x-rays allowed manipulation of the data to change the presentation of the image. One technique that has come into widespread use is **digital subtraction angiography (DSA)**, which was introduced commercially in 1980 (78). The technique usually involves injecting contrast medium into the veins and detecting the changes brought about by the contrast medium passing through the vascular structures of diagnostic interest (54;77). DSA can be used in diagnostic studies of arteries over the entire body, and can be useful in documenting such problems as atherosclerotic blockages of vessels. However, problems with artifacts from motion of the patient or internal organs have not been entirely solved, which has prevented DSA from living up to initial high expectations in the field of cardiovascular diagnosis.

During the last 30 years, **ultrasound imaging** has become one of the most widespread imaging techniques, and still may be the most rapidly spreading (36). Ultrasound did not develop as rapidly as CT scanning, in part because images were difficult to produce and interpret (61). However, improvements in the technology in the 1970s have led to rapid spread into many areas of medicine, especially in obstetrics, where it is used to image the fetus, uterus, and placenta within a pregnant woman. Ultrasound is based on the physics of sound rather than on ionizing radiation, and is therefore not associated with the known risks of such radiation, which makes it especially attractive for obstetric imaging. The basic technology of ultrasound imaging consists of a transducer that converts electrical signals into high frequency mechanical (sound) waves that are transmitted into the body. The echos from structures within the body are then received by the transducer and converted back into electrical signals. A processor then uses these signals to produce an image on a display monitor. Ultrasound can produce a two-dimensional, cross-sectional view of a body tissue or structure. The problem with ultrasound is that the sound waves do not easily penetrate bone or dense tissue, so it is mainly used in soft tissue parts of the body, such as the orbit of the eye, the heart, and the uterus. Ultrasound also does not reflect air or bowel gas, which means that no image is produced. A final problem is that ultrasound images are difficult to reproduce. Increasingly, ultrasound has used digital data, and it can now be incorporated as part of a digital system.

Another common imaging technology is made up of **nuclear medicine**, which uses radioactive tracers that are injected into the body. Such tracers were used as early as 1927. Early 'scans' entailed injection of a radioactive substance such as radioactive iodine that accumulated in one organ (the thyroid in the case of iodine) and scanning of the organ for radioactivity levels and for concentrations of radioactivity or 'cold spots' that might indicate pathological processes. In 1962 radionuclides were used to produce images of the heart (68). In a typical study, a radiopharmaceutical is injected into a resting or exercising patient and is distributed to tissues depending on its chemical and physical characteristics. Gamma radiation emitted by the radionuclide is measured externally by a detector. As indicated above, the detector can produce a picture directly, in analogue fashion. However, most systems now use digital methods. Tomographic techniques have also been applied to nuclear medicine to produce two-dimensional images (68). Nuclear medicine is widely available, but is not always integrated with departments of radiology. Positron Emission Tomography (PET) scanners, a technology in experimental use in a number of medical centers, is an advanced form of imaging using short-lived radionuclides that is also based on digital methods (71). The Netherlands presently has one PET scanner in operation in Groningen.

Another device producing digital images, the **magnetic resonance imaging (MRI) scanner**, was introduced in the late 1970s and is spreading into use as a diagnostic tool (35). At present, MRI uses signals from hydrogen atoms in the body to produce images of the internal structures of the body. Hydrogen atoms spin and have a polarity (that is, they act as small magnets). When placed in a strong static magnetic field, some of them align themselves with the field. A radio frequency (electromagnetic) field can then be applied at right angles to the static field, which causes the hydrogen atoms to precess (or 'wobble') in phase. When the radio field is turned off, the nuclei return to an equilibrium state, generating a signal with a similar radio frequency, which can be picked up by receiver coils. These signals can be used to construct images, using mathematical analysis and reconstruction done by computer. MRI produces images of cross-sections of the human body similar to those produced by computed tomography (CT) scanners (59). There are important differences, however. A CT image depicts the x-ray opacity of structures of the body. MRI images depict the density or even the chemical environment of hydrogen atoms. These properties of parts of the body are not necessarily correlated. MRI has several advantages. It gives a high contrast sensitivity in its images. It does not employ ionizing radiation as CT scanning and other imaging methods do. It is not necessary to inject potentially toxic contrast agents, as is often done with CT scanning, although the use of contrast agents may become widespread in the future. MRI allows choice of different imaging planes without moving the patient; CT scanning can only produce an image of one plane at a time, and some planes are not possible. Finally, images can be obtained from areas of the body where CT scanning fails to produce clear images (59). The Netherlands presently has 4 MRI devices, with a possibility of additional devices within the next year or so.

Thus, the field of radiology has changed dramatically since its inception, with a number of highly sophisticated technologies at its command. Indeed, many departments of radiology have changed their name to 'department of medical imaging' or something similar to reflect the change that has occurred. Changes will continue to be rapid in the future. It is estimated that 50 percent of images will be digital by the year 1990 (57;58)

Present Developments

Conventional radiology continues to be the predominant form of imaging. Images are stored in analog form on film. The physician responsible for interpretation of the studies examines a series of films. He reviews the images, mentally discards non-useful information, and concentrates on important features of the image. He may request further studies to produce additional information. He then arrives at an interpretation or diagnosis. The film is stored in a film jacket in an archive until it is needed again. This method of data handling has been historically successful, but has problems. It is labor-intensive, slow, and may not provide the most important information (47;49).

At the same time, conventional radiology has changed. About 20 percent of the work of the cardiology department is done with via image intensifier fluoroscopy. The image intensifier includes a monitor, so a digital output can be easily obtained.

It seems feasible to digitize all conventional radiology. Philips has found that x-ray plates can be read by laser-beam to produce digital data that can then be manipulated to improve the usefulness of the images. X-ray dose is reduced. Philips also has 3 years of experience with stimulated phosphor screens as a detector for the x-rays.

Widespread application of the digital imaging techniques, which now make up perhaps 20 percent of imaging procedures in larger hospitals (but only about 2-3 percent of data collected and stored), has given new important capabilities for making diagnosis. It has also led to new data handling problems (12). The digital data must also be stored; it must be accessible quickly in case of need; its distribution must be limited to those who have a right to it. To the present, most storage of digital images is on film, so the traditional system generally continues as before. At the same time, the new and less invasive imaging methods have led to an increased number of tests, which has complicated problems of storage and access (49). Film jackets cannot be used for several purposes simultaneously. Access to a film jacket is limited to a single user or single display site. Transfer of the film jacket from user to user takes time (21). Film jackets are sometimes lost and misplaced (58). A particular problem with patients who are acutely ill is that several different physicians may need to see an image within a short period of time, for example, when a patient is in an intensive care unit.

Digital imaging modalities can improve this process in certain ways (57). The supervising physician can alter the diagnostic procedure during its course in the case of MRI, CT scanning, and ultrasound. Prior images can be called back for examination while the patient is still available. The data collected can also be processed and manipulated to emphasize certain possibly abnormal features. This can make the diagnostic process more efficient, saving resources and avoiding excessive radiation dose to the patient. These characteristics, along with the potential speed of access and the possibility of easier storage, have led to proposals for fully digitized systems.

One of the greatest advantages of digital imaging is image processing (70). Because the image is based on numerical data, it can be manipulated by computer programs. Images can be enhanced by smoothing or sharpening them. Standard preprocessing techniques now include deblurring, outlining, noise reduction, filtering, and rejection of artifacts (44). Once the image has been preprocessed and is in the computer memory, it can be further processed. Picture processing usually involves, first, searching for objects of interest, and second, analyzing the objects of interest. For example, objects of interest can be digitized again in higher spatial resolution so that they are seen more clearly (44). In addition, digital processing in CT scanning and MRI makes the development of three-dimensional images possible.

Computer assisted imaging can also be integrated with radiotherapy in treatment planning. This has been called CART (computer aided radiotherapy) (51). In such a system, computer assisted imaging would be involved in localization of the tumor, treatment planning, simulation of the radiotherapy, and checking and confirming the therapy (27). Such systems do not yet exist. Since 1983, a NORDFORSK project, financed by the Nordic Industrial Fund and consisting of people representating radiophysics departments, radiotherapy departments, and industry, has been working on the design of such a system (22).

Another aspect of importance in digital systems is the electronic communication of images, teleradiology. In 1947, x-ray images were transmitted by phone lines for the first time. Now, electronic image transmission at high data rates is becoming increasingly common. Transmission media now include direct microwaves, satellite relay, and coaxial or fiberoptic cable (29). Images can be transmitted from remote sites to central location (for interpretation, for example) (49). An essential component of PACS will be data transmission within a department of radiology or within a hospital.

One problem with medical imaging at the present is the large amount of data collected on a patient. This strains the capabilities of radiologists and others to interpret the images. This problem could be solved - or partially solved - in the future by the use of expert systems for the interpretation of selected images (15;33;50). Computer assisted diagnostic systems have already been developed for a number of areas of medicine, and work on artificial intelligence seems certain to make better systems possible (4;13;63;79). With all of the data from a procedure in the computer, it would be a natural development to also have a computer interpretation of the data.

Up to the present, computer assisted medical imaging (or digital imaging) has been added to departments of radiology without changing them dramatically. Data are stored on film and these films are stored and retrieved just as x-ray films are.

In a department based entirely on digital systems, all imaging technologies would be integrated by one computerized system, with video consoles in the main department, consoles in other parts of the hospital or remote sites, transmission lines connecting sites, and computerized storage of the data both for short term recall and long term archiving (12;26). A full system with these characteristics has come to be called the **Picture Archiving and Communications System (PACS)**. No such system is now in operation, but several are in development. The possible advantages of such a system are detailed in the next sections. The technical aspects of such a system will only be described briefly. A number of excellent reviews of digital radiology and PACS are available (40;44;45;58;65;74). A number of useful articles and an extensive set of references may be found in

Hohne (43). The publications of the BAZIS group in Leiden give full information, both on general developments and on the situation in the Netherlands (2;53;72;73).

Necessary Technical Developments in PAC Systems

The essence of a PACS is that it is a system of stations interconnected by a network. The stations carry out key functions in medical imaging: acquisition stations, where the images are created by a diagnostic device in contact with a patient; display stations, where the images are selected and displayed; work stations, where images can be selected, displayed, manipulated, and annotated; and archives, where images can be stored for later recall and use (23;24;39;74;75) (see Figure 1). Such a total system would involve only images created in electronic form. It could be based only on the digital systems described above, but it might also involve the replacement of analogue systems such as conventional x-ray with digital systems. Conventional x-ray can be converted to digital form either by x-ray units that replace film with electronic detectors or by scanning the film with a reader to convert its data to numeric form. A number of such systems are now becoming available (30).

PACS has not developed as rapidly as some have predicted. One problem may be lack of a consensus on what problem PACS is intended to address. Another overall problem is the lack of a systematic view on how to realize a prototype system, with its many complexities, which has led to costly errors through 'trial and error' approaches (72;73). Developing a complete system requires technical developments in a number of areas, including both hardware and software areas. A full PACS has large mass storage requirements, and developments are needed in display set-up, image processing, and data compression (these issues are discussed further in the paragraphs to follow). Many hardware components are either not available or are too expensive. They also are not yet standardized, which leads to problems in trying to build up a system. Initial costs are high for a full prototype, but possible economic benefits seem most convincing when the system is complete (24). Another problem is that physicians, including radiologists, need to become accustomed to practicing in front of a video display device instead of a film viewbox. Radiologists have often not been involved in development of systems, which heightens their resistance (72). In addition, CRT images often are unsatisfactory, with poor spatial resolution, flicker, and other problems (24).

Figure 1 The concept of a PAC system

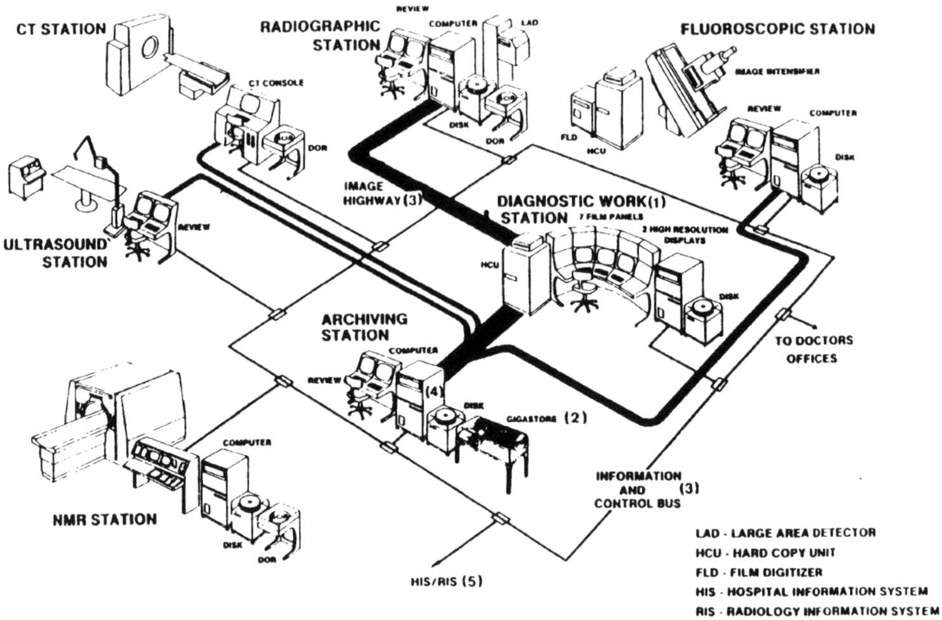

Source: Philips

Digital radiology gives an alternative for storage (41;65). Instead of a physical facility (perhaps a room in the basement) for the films, storage can be done on computer discs or magnetic tape, which must also be stored, but require far less space, although the space might need special physical conditions, so it might be more expensive. Digital storage has other differences from the conventional method. Some of the discs, at least, would need to be quickly available, but with present technology, a hospital might require as many as 20,000 discs to archive ten years of images. A conventional chest x-ray might require 50 times as much storage capacity on a disc as a CT scanner image (47). A high-resolution coronary angiogram with six injections of dye could generate nearly 2 billion bits of data (37). The size and availability of the computer and the type and number of discs are then key aspects to consider. Presently-available discs and tapes lack the capacity to store the amounts of data mentioned and to make them rapidly available. Laser or optical discs have a larger capacity, but even they do not solve the problem. A single laser disc may be able to store up to 10 billion bits of data per side. This means that one disc could store almost 10,000 images, but it still would only be able to handle 166 ordinary chest films (37). Data compression (see later) could partially solve this problem, but not completely.

Access to the stored information is also a critical issue (28;48). This information is necessary for patient care, so a certain amount of it must be 'on-line', or at least on readily accessible discs. It could be quite time consuming for a system to search for the appropriate disc and bring it on-line. A system based on discs would have to be hierarchical, with some discs quickly available and others available only after a time delay. One problem is that digital images are sought more often than film, perhaps because of the easier access (24).

Transmission of the data is another problem. All currently available methods are associated with a limited rate of transmission (37). Twisted pairs, for example (high quality telephone-type lines) are limited to about 1200 bytes per second. At that rate, it would take 3.48 hours to transmit the data in a single chest film. Broadband systems can transmit 1.25 Mbytes per second, and 50 to 250 channels can be used simultaneously; these systems can transmit the data on a standard chest film in about 1 second (37). Fiberoptic systems have the highest available rate of transmission, but are expensive.

Finally, the display device is obviously important, since the purpose is to produce information useful for diagnosis. It is important to make a distinction between work stations, where radiologists display images for processing, interpretation, and annotation, and display stations, where clinical physicians and others can see images but not process them. Presently available display devices cannot use all of the information on a conventional x-ray. In addition, display devices by different manufacturers have perceptual problems, in that the images produced can sometimes be interpreted differently, depending on the device. Still, display stations are generally within the limits of present technology and are not prohibitively expensive. Two levels of display device might be distinguished: 1) Some magnification is needed and some contrast so that the requestor can see the image. One might be available in each department, with perhaps 30-40 in a big hospital. 2) A video screen and frame grabber, where the information is needed for quick access and an overview. This kind of viewing station can be comparatively simple (53).

In contrast, work stations present enormous technical challenges (24;67). Lightboxes in present film reading rooms have space for eight or so chest radiographs, and display may be motor-driven, so that film can be changed in a second or two. Radiologists sometimes need very high resolution of the image and image processing capability, which means expensive systems. The speed of response is another problem, and although it is technically feasible to build systems that change as rapidly as the conventional lightbox systems, they are very expensive (24). Finally, work stations need to be ergonomic, that is, they must be comfortable and easy for a radiologist to use. How to design work stations to optimize use and interpretation of digital images is a developing art. Work is proceeding on all of these problems, including attempts to develop display devices capable of displaying an entire radiograph in high resolution form, but how rapidly satisfactory solutions can be found is not known.

An important issue in these systems is 'data compression' (2;25;46). A typical CT scanner image is made up of a 512 by 512 matrix of 'pixels' (picture elements) and it takes more than 5 minutes to transmit it by a telephone line. In a system being developed at the University of Kansas in the United States, the developers estimate that 1.2 million bits of data must be transmitted each second, just for their facility's imaging modalities (21). Data compression is of benefit for both data storage and data transmission.

Several manufacturers have systems that electronically compress the data to as little as one-thirtieth of the original amount (20;29). Hardware is now available that makes compression and decompression a rapid process. A few studies have been done showing that such data compression leads to images of lower quality. However, the implications of such reductions in image quality for correct interpretation of the pictures or for treatment guidance have been little studied (75). A critical question is if the image based on more data is clinically better. What is essential for correct diagnosis? New systems of data compression are being developed that may produce images of higher quality (62).

Another technological issue concerns conversion of x-rays to digital form (42). Devices are now available that can carry out such conversion, but since the amount of data in an analogue x-ray film is great, this necessarily involves data compression.

From the radiologist's point of view, a PACS must assist in the diagnostic interpretation of radiological images (38;67):

- it must allow fast access to all present-day images of the patient, as well as preceding images and reports;
- it must allow simple and rapid placement and ordering of images;
- it must provide adequate spatial and contrast resolution of the images;
- it must be simple to operate and ergonomic for the radiologist.

It would also be desirable for the PACS to be connected to a broader hospital information system (HIS) so that the radiologist would have access to other data on the patient (14).

A series of steps are necessary to develop a fully integrated PAC system. One scenario might be as follows. First, present-day digital imaging must be made compatible with the PACS. This will require a standard interface for data transfer. Then PACS consoles will be tried out in demonstration sites and they will be modified based on radiologist reactions. Next, partial PAC systems will integrate digital procedures such as CT scanning or nuclear medicine into the routine of a radiology department. These systems will be limited by available storage capacity and limited ability to transfer images. When future communication networks involving computers allow rapid transfer of large amounts of data, a total departmental PAC system can be implemented. The final step cannot be expected before 1995 (38).

The possible advantages of PACS are detailed in Sections 3 and 4.

Developing a PACS: The Role of Industry and Research Groups

Development of a fully-integrated PAC system obviously requires industrial involvement. Neither the R&D support nor the technical expertise is available outside the industrial sector. The optimal situation involves cooperation between industry, research groups, and one or more hospitals (18).

Attempts to develop a PAC system could be said to be either 'bottom-up' or 'top-down' (72). A bottom-up approach would involve automation of the image handling by some type of PACS within a department of radiology. This could lead to a fully functioning departmental PACS, in which the user, with support from the referring physicians (to whom the images are delivered) and clinical physicist's, specifies the functional requirements and is able to gradually bring about changes in the local organization. The top-down approach involves hospital-wide integration of a PACS with an existing Hospital Information System (HIS) (76). This will cost much more, raises many more technical problems, requires more personnel, and raises many problems of coordination and interfacing, but is expected to result in a full-grown, flexible, and powerful PAC system (72). Both types of approach are necessary in a combined effort (40).

The involvement of Philips in developing computer assisted medical images integrated into the Hospital Information System in Utrecht developed by BAZIS will be described below (72). Components of the prototype PACS are made by Raytel, a U.S. firm in which Philips owns a part. Philips also has a radiological information system (RIS) on the market, and it could eventually market a PACS integrated into that system. The first step, however, will be to couple the PACS to the BAZIS information system, including the radiology subsystem. Philips has its most active involvement through its Hamburg branch, and it is supported by the German Ministry for Research and Technology. It is working on developing a Medical Archiving and Communication System (MARCOM) for the general hospital. Philips has also developed a relationship with the American Telephone and Telegraph Company (AT&T), a major communication company, because of its interest in more general applications of video communication systems.

Siemens is a European company quite interested in PACS. Siemens formed an advanced development group in Erlangen, Germany in 1984 to develop laboratory demonstration PACS components in order to understand problems of maintaining very large data bases of imaging and presenting them to health care providers in efficient ways (38;39). Siemens anticipates that chest radiography will become digital in the future, which will mean that the department of radiology will be more than 50 percent digital (in numbers of examinations) even without further developments. Siemens is cooperating with the Department of Radiology, Catholic University, Nijmegen, and others, including the University Hospital in Montpellier, on PACS-related issues. In British Columbia, Canada, the Ministry of Health is supporting the development and evaluation of a full PACS in Victoria General Hospital in collaboration with Siemens. The Canadian group expects a fully operational PAC system by 1990 (16).

A number of European groups are working on PACS. These include the Vrije Universiteit in Brussels; the DIMI project group at the University Hospital, Nantes; and the SIRENE project at the University Hospital of Rennes (in cooperation with CGR and others).

In the United States, there is no working PACS or PACS prototype. U.S. efforts are described in detail elsewhere (6;56). The following institutes, among others, are actively working in the area, all using small computers (72;73):

- the University of North Carolina in Chapel Hill and the North Carolina Memorial Hospital;
- the Hospital of the University of Pennsylvania in Philadelphia;
- the University of Arizona Medical Center in Tucson (collaborating with Toshiba);
- the University of Kansas Medical Center in Kansas City (initially sponsored by NCR Corporation, which has since withdrawn) (23);
- the Mallinckrodt Institute of Radiology in St. Louis.

de Valk and Boekee (72) comment that these institutes seem to lack an overall system philosophy as a basis for PACS design, development, and introduction into daily clinical practice. They are working on a 'trial and error' basis, focusing on different PACS components, mostly based on the equipment already available.

Other U.S. hospitals are also working on PACS development, generally only on subcomponents of a system, such as a totally digitized nuclear medicine system (23):

- Beth Israel Hospital in Boston;
- George Washington University Medical Center, Washington, D.C.;
- Middlesex General University Hospital, New Brunswick, N.J.;
- New York Hospital, Cornell Medical Center, New York, N.Y. (in collaboration with Technicare Corporation);
- New York University Medical Center, New York, N.Y.;
- St. Luke's Hospital, Milwaukee, Wisconsin;
- UCLA Medical Center, Los Angeles, California;
- University of Connecticut Health Center, Framington, Connecticut;
- Veterans Administration Medical Center, Milwaukee, Wisconsin.

Drew (23) gives a list of companies, mostly U.S. based, interested in developing PACS or components for PACS.

In Japan, the major activity is not in hospitals and research institutes but in industry. Japan is making a major investment in the development of new technologies, especially those related to communications and data processing. At the 5th Symposium on Medical Imaging Technology in Japan in July 1986 thirteen papers were presented by manufacturers, and more than 12 Japanese companies actively support the Japan Society of PACS. It is anticipated that the Japanese will have advanced products, including a full PACS, and that many European companies will only be able to function in this market by marketing Japanese products or manufacturing them under license (55).

Overall, Europe is behind in hardware, but only about two years. Europe is probably further behind in software developments (72). The overall European investment in telecommuncations and data processing is small in comparison with that of the United States and Japan.

Useful information on international efforts in developing PACS may be found in the EuroPACS newsletter, published by the BAZIS group in Leiden. EuroPACS is a voluntary organization of cooperation between research and development groups from universities, hospitals, and industries of the countries of Europe (6;72).

Activities in the Netherlands Concerning PACS

The Netherlands has a rather well-organized effort to develop and test a functional PACS. The effort involves the hospital information system and data processing expertise of the BAZIS Organization group with its headquarters in Leiden; the University Hospital in Utrecht; Philips; and the image processing and computer expertise of the University of Technology in Delft. The effort has been partially funded by the Ministry of WVC.

Leiden started following developments in PACS in 1984 and wrote a report, sponsored by WVC, on what PACS could mean. The system envisaged was based on the hospital information system, used by 27 hospitals in the Netherlands, including all academic hospitals except one. At the end of 1984, WVC sponsored the development of a software simulation of the PACS (76). Such aspects of the system as bottlenecks, through-put, and queuing were modelled (53). (Leiden is also supported by the Dutch Science Foundation, ZWO.)

As for the University Hospital in Utrecht, it is a member of the BAZIS Organization and uses its hospital information system (40). It has all established digital imaging modalities (CT scanning, digital substraction angiography, nuclear medicine, magnetic resonance imaging, ultrasound). Beginning in December 1983, the hospital began to consider going further into digitized systems. The interest of the hospital focused on patient care. The presence of an interdepartmental Working Group on Image Processing in Medicine provided a good basis of collaboration among different departments, including radiology, nuclear medicine, and computer science. Furthermore, the Department of Nuclear Medicine has been digital since 1975 and had gradually developed a 'mini-PACS.' Finally, the University Hospital has a long tradition of cooperation with Philips in radiology. Since 1978, it has been Philips' main site for examining applications of CT scanning and image processing in digital substraction angiography. Philips is now supporting a three year effort in clinical and scientific research involving MRI at the Hospital.

Philips is deeply involved in digital imaging, with CT scanning and MRI systems on the international market. Philips also has a computerized radiology information system. However, Philips was interested in exploring the possibilities of merging digital systems with a comprehensive hospital information system.

In February 1986, a contract was signed involving Leiden, Philips, and Utrecht for three years, with the aim of developing a prototype PACS, connected to the hospital information system. There are two parties formally: 1) the consortium of BAZIS organization, Philips, and the University Hospital, Utrecht, with the University of Technology in Delft as the main subcontractor to BAZIS; and 2) WVC funding the bulk of the evaluation work.

The decision was made to first develop the system for one wing of internal medicine, involving 15 beds. For all patients in those beds, all images will be processed digitally. The Utrecht system includes a viewing station, a filing system (one optical disc), and a scanning system. It is similar to the Raytel (U.S.) system (Raytel is 20 percent Philips owned). The equipment was installed during late 1986. A digitizer will convert all regular x-rays. The filing system will probably be based on 4 optical recorder discs. An ergonomically-designed digital reading room has been set up to cope with the patient load. In this room, located in the center of the Department, an image viewing system for CT, DSA, and MRI are combined with the PACS viewing station. The digitized system will be connected to the hospital information system during the summer of 1987 by BAZIS. The image viewing system is a 6 screen box with 1024 by 1024 resolution each. Evaluation of the system will include comparison to two reference or control groups, on other medical wards.

The pilot study will be needed to advise WVC and Philips how to proceed. After 1 year, the project should give WVC rough indications of costs and benefits, and after 3 years, a more comprehensive evaluation should have been completed.

It will probably take at least 10 years to have good comprehensive products, but there will probably be valuable by-products, in the design of high tech equipment, for example.

The goal in the project is to have a long-term involvement in digital imaging. Philips obviously wants a commercial system of value in a working hospital. Utrecht wants to demonstrate benefits to patients at a reasonable cost. Leiden wants to test the feasibility of integrating image handling with a comprehensive hospital information system. And Delft wishes to assist in developing a workable system within the Netherlands.

Early in 1987, the Ministry of WVC granted the funding to allow the next steps in the combined development of the prototype system.

Section 2 – Health Care Implications of Computer Assisted Medical Imaging

Computer assisted medical imaging has made new and dramatic diagnostic procedures available. These have had a variety of consequences both for the health care system and for patients. Consequences range from effects on health to changes in health care delivery patterns. Some of these consequences may intensify as computer assisted imaging spreads and PAC systems develop.

This Section will discuss the implications of computer assisted imaging for the health system, excluding the issue of financial costs. Possible effects of PACS will be mentioned, but at present no data are available on those potential effects. The next Section will discuss the benefits of computer assisted imaging, focusing on PACS, in relation to its costs.

A diagnostic technology can be evaluated at several different levels (see Table 1). The policy maker tends to be most interested in the highest levels, in particular the question of societal efficacy. The physician is most interested in effects on health.

Implications of Computer Assisted Imaging for Health

It is difficult to evaluate the impacts of a diagnostic technology on health. In general, diagnostic technologies have been evaluated technically; occasionally, their precision has been evaluated; they have seldom been evaluated for their effects on health. A full evaluation of a diagnostic technology would include studies on all medical conditions or indications for diagnosis, with evidence of the impact of the particular diagnostic procedure.

In some cases, computer assisted medical imaging has been shown to be important for health outcomes. For example, CT scanning of the brain has replaced invasive exploratory neurosurgical procedures in cases of head injury, and may be assumed to be of health benefit in such cases (3;60). However, demonstrating effects of a diagnostic procedure on health outcome is very difficult (1;11;34). In particular, this is because improving health depends on the availability and application of an effective therapy.

Table 1 Levels at which diagnostic imaging techniques may be assessed

Level of the measurement	Typical output measures
Level 1 Image efficacy	Quality of image resolution
Level 2 Image and observer efficacy	Percentage yield of abnormal cases: percentage correct diagnoses; sensitivity specificity
Level 3 Diagnostic efficacy	Change in order of clinicians diagnostic considerations
Level 4 Management efficacy (therapeutic decision-making)	Percentage change in therapeutic protocol percentage change in appropriate therapy
Level 5 Patient outcome efficacy	Survival rates; percentage cures; morbidity measures; reduced worry of patient and family
Level 6 Societal efficacy (or utility)	Dollars added to GNP; age-adjusted survival rates

Source: reference 54

It seems unlikely that fully digitized systems can be demonstrated to have an important effect on human health. Therefore, evaluations must concentrate on other effects that are easier to demonstrate.

Improved diagnosis. An improved diagnosis should, in certain circumstances, lead to better treatment. Thus, it may be generally assumed that improving diagnosis is a worthwhile aim.

Computer assisted imaging gives the interested health care provider the ability to make better diagnoses for a number of reasons. In some cases, such as brain tumors, diagnoses can be made that were difficult, if not impossible, to make before. The introduction of CT scanning, for example, lead to a dramatic reduction in the number of invasive procedures such as neurosurgery used to diagnose lesions in the brain due to trauma (60). Although this capability has not been shown to lead directly to improved health outcomes, it seems evident that the avoidance of dangerous procedures is a worthwhile outcome. Computer assisted imaging also gives the ability to manipulate the image so that abnormalities can be seen more clearly and more exactly localized. This, too, should lead to some improvements in health outcome, although they might be small in the aggregate.

Computer assisted imaging makes it possible to make three-dimensional images. The implications of such images are being explored. They could be quite useful in a few areas, such as evaluation of inborn abnormalities, orthopedics, trauma, and neurosurgery. Such imaging is now starting to be used in designing and manufacturing prostheses (computer aided manufacturing, or CAM), especially where a good fit will improve mechanical strength, as in total hip joint replacement.

Computer assisted imaging can guide other diagnostic procedures, such as needle biopsies (60;61).

An important development that has spread since the introduction of CT scanning is to use imaging to guide therapeutic procedures. For example, abscesses can be drained by a needle after they are localized on an image. Imaging is used to guide procedures done by catheters, such as balloon dilatation of blood vessels (see report on laser treatment of coronary artery disease, another case study in this project). Drugs can also be installed in certain parts of the body by guided needle (60;61).

X-ray dose. A major orientation in technological developments in the field of diagnostic imaging has been to reduce the dose of ionizing radiation delivered to people, since this radiation is associated with risks (27). These efforts have been historically successful, through such innovations as control of the spread of the x-ray beam, development of image intensifiers, and ability to reconstruct and manipulate an image through computers. Also, the rapid growth of ultrasound imaging and magnetic resonance imaging is in part because they are probably safer than imaging based on x-rays or other ionizing radiation.

One reason for excessive radiation dose to patients is repeat films because of poor quality x-ray images. Image quality can also be enhanced by image processing, which is not possible with film. Some evidence is available that computer assisted medical imaging can reduce radiation dose to the patient (5;52).

Improved access to images. Sometimes it is critically important to have rapid access to images, as in emergency situations. A patient might have an abnormality on an image, for example, and only comparison with an older image could indicate if it was new or not. It can sometimes be difficult to gain access to x-ray films from the archives. Sometimes it takes hours or longer to find or access an image in the present system, because of the limited number of copies, multiple archives, overloaded archive personnel, lost or wrongly placed images, or loaned images. Computer assisted imaging might improve access. In particular, images can no longer be lost with such systems (although discs can possibly be lost). Furthermore, multiple copies can be easily made, increasing availability.

Computer assisted imaging could be particularly important when the patient is in a remote site. It could even be the case that no one with expertise in interpreting images was available. The image could be transmitted to a central site for interpretation. Such interpretation might be life-saving in some instances, but no data are available to indicate how often such a development would be of benefit.

The problem in this area is the state of the art. Problems of access and rapid transmission of images still need to be solved. The BAZIS group is carrying out research on these problems.

Possible Implications of PAC Systems for the Organization of Health Care

Effects of PAC systems are speculative. The purpose of this part is to suggest some implications that might be evaluated in the future.

For the physician, the first concern will be that the diagnostic process is just as efficient (if not more so) than it was under conventional methods. Since conventional radiology is now highly automated in many ways, this may be difficult to demonstrate. At present, images are available to the physician in three ways:

1. in emergencies, the images are sent immediately, and a report follows;
2. in ordinary situations, images and report are sent later, perhaps the next day;
3. in certain situations, and at the request of the clinical physician, consultations are held between referring physicians and radiologists to discuss diagnosis and therapy (27).

Some medical imaging services are only available in central locations, while others are quite diffused. CT scanners and MRI devices are generally quite centralized, in academic hospitals. Nuclear medicine is more widely diffused, but is only available through departments of radiology or medical imaging. Conventional x-ray tends to be centralized into such departments, but can also be available at the primary care level and in remote sites. Ultrasound is widely distributed throughout the system.

One possibly important effect of PACS is that clinical physicians must now often visit the radiology department to examine the images and discuss them with the radiologist. With computer-assisted imaging, it is possible to transmit the image to any site with the appropriate equipment and discuss it by telephone. This could result in a significant time saving for the clinical physician. However, the possibly negative implications of less face-to-face consultation between physicians needs to be considered as well. In addition, the ready access of other patient data through the Hospital Information System (HIS) may more than counter-balance such implications.

PACS can tie together different parts of the health care system. One hospital could, for example, serve the imaging needs of a region. Experts could be available for interpretation of images taken in smaller or less specialized hospitals. Primary care centers, too, could be tied into such a system, so that diagnosis by images could be made more effectively in clinics. This area is called teleradiology.

Computer assisted medical imaging and PACS have important potential implications for the health care delivery system. They automate the diagnostic process further. (The physician is already able to supervise multiple procedures at the same time from a central point.) One task that has been envisioned is the supervision of radiotherapy, through the integration of radiotherapy and imaging (51). Another possibility is to integrate digital imaging with neurosurgery through a surgical robot with a vision system, enabling high-precision surgical operations (27). The radiologist of the future will probably be much more involved in intervention, and may also find new demands in the diagnostic process. One problem is the proliferation of information. Someone must interpret this information to make a diagnosis. The person who interprets medical images in the future will need to understand more about such areas of physiology, biochemistry, and other aspects of biological functioning. Expert systems, as mentioned above, may be helpful.

Ultimately, the implications of PACS are to tie health care sites together into one system. The health care system has developed as centralized, tertiary care institutions with collections of specialists and expensive technology. This type of system has in part developed because of needs for communication and consultation between specialists. More efficient methods of communication could end this need. Many kinds of information besides images easily can be transferred by such systems: laboratory results, clinical consultations, patient record information, and so forth.

Acceptance of PACS by Radiologists and Other Physicians

The radiologist is the physician who must accept digital imaging and computer assistance, including PACS. Any system must, then, be acceptable to the radiologist. Radiologists have already accepted computer assisted imaging methods such as CT scanning. But when imaging processing and computer storage of data are added, the radiologist's role changes.

Any system must be simple to operate; present systems are not 'user-friendly.' It must also be ergonomic. That is, it must be easy to operate physically; it must not put inappropriate physical strains on the operator; the images must be presented in such a way that they do not cause undue eye strain. As mentioned previously, present display devices have problems and work station design is not yet optimal. The investment by a physician, especially in time required to become familiar with a system, can be a problem in acceptance.

An important aspect of physician acceptance concerns the speed of retrieval of images. Physicians will not accept a system that cannot produce information needed for optimal patient care when it is needed. It may also be necessary to somehow differentiate images that are 'on-line' because they may be medically needed, and images that are on disc and accessible after some delay. System simulation as carried out by the Imagis Project can be useful in developing retrieval systems.

Training of Radiologists and Others

Developing and using PACS is a highly interdisciplinary activity, involving experts in information technology, clinical physics, engineering, robotics, and artificial intelligence, as well as physicians. Training programs need to take this into account, teaching different technical languages, for example. It could be beneficial to have interdisciplinary training programs as well.

Using technology such as computer assisted medical imaging equipment requires more skills than are usually called for in health care. The images themselves need to be validated. The technical quality of the equipment must be assured. The use of the equipment is also important. Physicians and others need to understand the limitations of the equipment, especially in terms of specificity and sensitivity. These are growing problems because of the flood of information. All of these aspects need to be part of specific training of those using the equipment. X-ray technicians and nurses are particularly important in this field, because it is they who generally carry out the routine imaging procedures and thereby influence image quality.

However, specific training in the use of equipment is often neglected at the present (27).

If PACS becomes entirely developed and accepted, it will change many aspects of medical diagnosis. Obviously, training programs must react to these changes. Ultimately, acceptance of PACS by radiologists will depend very much on the training that they have had.

Archiving

An important issue in computer-assisted medical imaging concerns archiving diagnostic images. Images (including conventional x-rays) are archived for years. In many countries, such archiving is required by law, perhaps for 10 years (27). Saving the images gives a basis for subsequent evaluation of the patient. More important from the legal point of view, the image gives documentation concerning what was actually done.

Traditionally, x-ray films have been archived in a physical facility and stored in a film jacket. Multiple films could be included in this jacket. However, in complex institutions, or in patients with a large number of films, more complicated methods of storage have been used, increasing space requirements and costs. In these systems, all x-rays films have been saved.

Computer assisted imaging gives an alternative for storage. Instead of a physical facility (perhaps a room in the basement), storage can be done, for example, on computer discs. This could save money and be more efficient in other ways (see next Section).

With the growing volume of information, selection of which images to save may become a critical issue. However, who is to decide which images are important for the future? What are the legal ramifications of not saving images? Committees of clinicians, administrators, lawyers, ethicists, and lay people may be required to develop guidelines for such a case.

Access and Confidentiality

The availability of medical images, whether conventional or digital, is subject to standards of privacy and confidentiality. Computer-assisted images raise new problems of privacy different from those faced in conventional systems. Conventional x-rays, being physical objects, could in theory be collected, transported, and stored, with little risk to confidentiality. Only those with documented reasons to need to see the films are allowed access. In reality, confidentiality has been a continuing problem in conventional systems. One problem has been the complexity of determining who should have the right to access, and when. For example, images are not usually freed to the clinician until the radiologist has checked their quality and made an interpretation.

Computer assisted images, being accessible by telephone wire and computer, raise problems already familiar with computerized Hospital Information Systems (HIS). They require safeguards. Many clinical physicians will review images in their ward or clinic situation. This requires retrieval systems and view boxes. Access must be relatively simple, so that physicians will use the system (47). However, easy access makes the problem of confidentiality more difficult. The normal method of control of such data is to have passwords or user-computer dialogues that require the entry of information before privileged patient information can be obtained. However, even a simple password system delays access and may not be acceptable to physicians. Technological developments such as magnetic cards or chip cards might solve this problem by providing automatic identification and access limitation.

This problem is even more acute in systems that are integrated into hospital information systems. Ultimately, such integration will become more common. The integration of data from different sources can improve diagnosis and therapy. But this also means that very sensitive data may be available to a wide range of health care providers (47).

Legislation to protect patient privacy is lagging in this field because of rapid technological developments (27). In the Netherlands, however, it has received a great deal of attention. Computerized systems have generally done well in protecting patient confidentiality.

Section 3 – A Framework for Evaluating PAC Systems

The main issue for policy making in the evaluation of PACS tends to be that of societal efficacy. In other words, the policy maker wishes to know how much benefit has been achieved for how much cost (10). This question cannot be answered in the case of PAC systems. There is no existing PAC system, so no empiric evaluation has been done. Evaluations of sub-parts of such systems have only just begun.

As indicated in the previous Section, benefits are difficult to evaluate in this case. Practically speaking, evaluations will not be able to address the issue of whether diagnostic imaging as currently practiced is in itself worthwhile. While some feel that PACS will ultimately have important effects on health, these possibilities are speculative at the moment. Costs of medical images at present can be estimated, but future costs are difficult to predict, especially for PACS.

The question still remains, how to evaluate the consequences of computer assisted medical imaging. In this Section, suggestions will be given for evaluating the field of computer assisted medical imaging, concentrating on financial costs (26). Table 2 outlines potential costs and benefits that might ultimately be evaluated. It seems unlikely, however, that PACS will spread unless the cost to the system is small. In other words, can the savings from PACS offset the investments needed?
An important issue that must be settled in the years to come is whether a total integrated PACS is truly feasible technically. It appears that it is, but, as indicated in the previous section, many technical issues remain to be solved.

Financial Costs

The dominant issue, assuming solution of the technological problems, is costs. The capital investments required could be large. For example, a 700 bed university hospital might require a total of 2000 optical disks annually to store its film and digital images, at a present cost as high as US$700 each (37). However, this cost will fall rapidly. Presently available 12 inch disks cost $US340 in the

Table 2 Potential costs and benefits of a change to digital imaging

Costs	Benefits
1. Additional capital costs (radiology equipment, computers building alterations)	1. Savings in materials (e.g. film, darkroom supplies)
2. Re-training of staff	2. Savings in capital costs (e.g. darkroom and equipment, film storage space)
3. Additional radiologist time in image manipulation and interpretation	3. Savings in technician and radiologist time in image production (leading to reduction in staff or re-deployment to other useful duties)
4. Additional maintenance costs (e.g. on computers)	4. Savings in hospitalization (thereby allowing beds to be closed or re-deployed)
	5. Health benefits and higher patient utility, in terms of reduced invasiveness of procedures and fewer radiation-induced tumours
	6. Savings in patients' time costs and (possibly) lost production
plus, if the system variables change:	
5. Costs of extra diagnostic procedures resulting from the removal of the "gatekeeper" effects of risk or need for hospital admission	7. Benefits (in health terms, or in terms of resource savings from the extra clinical procedures performed
6. Costs of extra clinical procedures arising from these extra diagnostic procedures	

Source: reference 23

Netherlands; this price is expected to fall to US$125 by 1991. Smaller disks and erasable disks will also appear, and their price will fall even lower.

As mentioned above, the entire hospital or health care system can be computerized. The computerization of the health care system has many advantages, and the costs cannot all be allocated to digital imaging. For example, better management information will generally improve patient care. This makes cost evaluation particularly difficult.

Frameworks for evaluating financial costs have been developed (23;26). These need to be applied to real, developing systems.

In this section, rough calculations on costs will be presented for illustrative purposes. This has the danger of leading one to assume that these costs will remain fixed, when in fact the field is changing rapidly technologically. However, without illustrative cost calculations, one cannot understand the importance of this issue for the health care system. In fact, if a full PACS were available, its purchase would be a large commitment for any hospital to undertake; for an entire society or health care system, the investment is truly enormous.

Drew (23) estimated annual costs for a 500 bed community hospital, including only the digital modalities. In this hospital, a daily number of 2364 standard picture frames are created. A standard picture frame uses the number of bytes needed for one image with the resolution and gray scale characteristics of an ultrasound image (512 by 512 by 1 = 0.25 megabytes). Of those 2364 standard pictures, 720 would be created by ultrasound, 24 by nuclear medicine, 820 by computerized tomography, 650 by digital subtraction studies, and 150 by magnetic resonance imaging. This set of digital modalities would create approximately 620 megabytes of new data daily. This production reflects actual average image production per bed in the United States.

The PAC system would consist of 6 work stations to enable radiologists to display, process, interpret, and annotate images, and 42 read-only display stations to be located mainly in nurses' stations, but also in intensive care units, operating rooms, emergency rooms, outpatient departments, and imaging departments. The requirements for work stations present enormous technical challenges. Costs per working station are estimated at US$250,000 on the basis of systems developed by Gould Inc., Imaging and Graphics Division. Display stations are nearly within the state of the art and are costed at US$5000.

Images would be stored in a short- and a long-term term archive. The short-term archive could consist of a multiple optical or magnetic disk drive or an optical disk 'jukebox' containing 100 optical disks. In this short-term archive the data of 10 days production of images (620 megabytes a day) are contained, supplemented with 50 percent for images of historical records of some patients. The capacity of the short-term archive is 9400 megabytes.

Costs of the short-term archive are derived from the price of the optical disk 'jukebox' offered by Raytel Medical Systems, costing about US$400,000.

The long-term archive would have the capacity to store the data of 1250 working days of 620 megabytes per day image production. For this a capacity of 775,000 megabytes would be needed, which presumably could be provided by two optical tape drivers and a microcomputer to manage the data base. The long-term archive would require 16 Drexon optical tape reels of 50,000 megabytes each to hold 1250 days of image data. The optical tape drivers would cost about US$200,000 and the microcomputer US$50,000. Both the facilities for the short- and the long-term archive would have to be available twice for the sake of reliability.

The hypothetical PAC system would need to be equipped with interfaces to adapt the data produced by the five image- creating departments (US$300,000) and with a communication system (US$300,000).

Nearly 70 percent of the annual costs of this hypothetical PAC system would be capital costs. The estimated capital costs are specified in Table 3.

The capital cost in this example is US$3.6 million. Assuming that capital costs are amortized in 5 years, that maintenance costs (including system analysts, programmers and technicians) amount to 5 percent of capital costs, that for consumables US$70,000 must be budgeted, and that a staff of 4 operators is needed to run the system, total annual costs of this PAC system, limited to digital modalities, amounts to just over US$1 million per year.

Table 3. Estimated capital costs for a PAC System integrating the digital imaging modalities, US Dollars

Work stations, 6 at US$250,000	US$ 1.5 million
Display stations 42 at US$5,000	0.2
Short-term archive 2 at US$425,000	0.8
Long-term archive 2 at US$250,000	0.5
Interfaces	0.3
Communication system	0.3

	US$ 3.6 million

While this might be considered a reasonable cost estimate for purposes of illustration, it does not include estimates for the cost of retraining staff (a one-time cost), possible additional radiologist time in image manipulation and interpretation, costs of extra diagnostic procedures that could result, and costs of extra clinical procedures arising from extra diagnostic procedures (26). A complete cost analysis would either include these variables or would present evidence that they were not significant.

The value of these estimates is not in the specifics. The specifics need to be confirmed in actual practice. Anyone interested can generate alternative estimates based on different assumptions. The value of the estimates is in the framework that they present for thinking about costs of the system.

Is the Investment Worth It?

As emphasized earlier, PACS may have other benefits than those of efficiency. However, in this Section, possible financial benefits are the focus.

The aspects of the evaluation that are most measurable are at the top of Table 2, and include such factors as savings in capital costs for cameras, darkroom, and storage space (21), savings in consumables associated with film, and savings in staff time because of increased efficiency. Also, fewer archive personnel might be required.

In addition, there are other possible savings that should be examined (23):

- reduction in lost and misplaced film and reports;
- reduction in retakes because of the ability to manipulate images;
- improved diagnostic accuracy because of image processing and ability to associate other clinical data with image data;
- faster diagnosis, with possible shorter length of stay;
- improved use of alternative facilities, such as day surgery, because of better diagnostic capabilities;
- increased efficiency of departmental operations.

An important possible saving is from the ability to transmit images from one site to another. For example, teleradiology systems used to transmit x-rays images between clinics and small hospitals and between small hospitals and large hospitals with radiology departments, seem to be cost-saving because the radiologist does not need to travel to remote sites to interpret x-rays. The same saving may be possible within a hospital, if a clinical physician does not need to go to the radiology department for a consultation with an expert.

Finally, it should not be forgotten that the ultimate aim is improvement in health. If radiation dosage to patients could be reduced, this is a clear benefit. Likewise, risky invasive diagnostic procedures, such as the injection of contrast materials, might be reduced. Both of these outcomes are measureable. Improvements in the diagnostic process, leading to improved therapy and health outcome, however, will generally be extremely difficult to document because of the complexity of the procedures involved and the fact that present capabilities are already high.

Answering the question as to whether PAC systems are worth it or not probably will lead many, including policy makers, to ask if such systems can pay for themselves through such factors as the first three in Table 2. The first question is whether digital diagnostic imaging allows the same diagnostic objectives to be met at less cost. The second question concerns the situation if the costs increase, either because costs are higher with digital imaging or because the quantity of the services provided increases, and whether this increase is associated with any demonstrable benefits in patient outcome or benefit (26). The answer to these questions is not known.

Drew (23) has estimated direct annual savings from installation of a PACS, to accompany his estimate of US$1 million costs for a fully integrated system. He estimates savings of US40,000 in capital costs, US$20,000 in maintenance costs, US$80,000 a year in consumables (especially x-ray film), and US$60,000 a year in staff savings (those previously required to manage the film archive). The total direct saving is then estimated at US$200,000. He concludes from this analysis that PACS are not economic at this time. He notes that this conclusion is related to the fact that available equipment is not optimal and is very expensive. This underlines the need for further technological developments.

At the same time, the more indirect costs enumerated could be highly significant. If the average length of stay in the hospital could be reduced half a day, for example, the saving would be large. Thus, potential indirect savings from PAC systems overshadow direct savings.

Drew (23) also notes that this conclusion applies only to a complete, integrated, institutional PACS. Smaller component systems may be already cost saving. PACS for nuclear medicine are available for less than US$100,000 and save more than they cost in the cost of film, film processing, and storage.

Conclusion

The most important question for policy is whether PACS are cost-effective or not. The question cannot be answered at the present.

There is no fully integrated, comprehensive PACS in operation. No direct evaluation can be done. Much technical development lies ahead.

A tentative conclusion can be reached that a fully comprehensive PACS would not pay for itself at this moment (66). However, the field is changing rapidly technologically. Hardware prices will surely decrease, while at the same time, available technology will become more suitable for PACS. This underscores not only the importance of further technological developments, but also of ongoing evaluation.

Section 4 – International Issues in Computer Assisted Imaging

As it was described in Volume I from the project, medical technology is an international issue. Health-related research and development is carried out internationally, and investments are spread widely over the world. Much technology is developed and marketed by the multinational industry. And technology assessment in health care is developing as an international activity to deal with these international aspects of technology development and diffusion.

In this Section, only international aspects specific to computer assisted medical imaging and PACS will be discussed.

Industry sales

The worldwide sales of diagnostic imaging equipment were estimated to be about US$4 billion in 1983. This amount is still growing relatively rapidly, and is expected to reach more than US$8 billion in 1988 (59). The most rapidly growing fields are digital x-ray and magnetic resonance imaging (27). The three largest companies are General Electric, Siemens, and Philips. These three companies produce the whole range of diagnostic imaging products. All are actively involved in developing PACS.

These figures do not include PACS, which had a world market in 1983 of about US$90 million (27). Economic analyses predict little impact on market sales of PACS by 1988.

Almost no company has the capability of producing all components for computer assisted imaging devices. For example, most of the magnets used in MRI devices are produced by Oxford Instruments and Intermagnetics (27). The utilization of sub-contractors is very common in this field because of its complexity. This means that growth in the field of computer assisted imaging will involve a large number of companies, both large and small.

International standards

A major problem in PACS is that there is no internationally-accepted standard for coding images for storage and transmission or for transmitting them (a communication protocol). Equipment is generally not compatible. This means that large companies are at a considerable advantage, since they are able to interconnect their own products. However, all companies use computer hardware that is not produced by them, so a common system would be beneficial to all in some ways (27).

Digital data transfer among devices with different data formats requires interface devices to translate formats and meet other requirements for compatibility (23). However, the designers of such devices must know the details of data format in the device on each side of the interface. In practice, it is necessary for the manufacturer to disclose such details, which they may not be willing to do. Even if they do, interface devices are not entirely satisfactory (23).

Most manufacturers and national standardization organizations have supported Open System Interconnection (OSI), which is being developed by the International Organization for Standardization (ISO).

In addition, the American College of Radiology (ACR) and the National Electrical Manufacturers Association (NEMA) in the United States are working together to prepare a standard (27). This standard is compatible with the ISO standards, but is limited to data exchange across an interface. Thus, further standards are necessary to develop a complete network (23). The ACR-NEMA group plans to continue to develop on system standards, but years of work are required. In addition, the standard will only apply to new devices and not to the large number of devices already in use. In Europe, ECMA is also working on developing standards, but these are not being developed in cooperation with radiologists. European efforts to develop standards could be expanded. At any rate, the next years of designing PAC systems will require the developer to face the problem of interfacing existing devices with the system.

Standards for equipment are absolutely required if smaller companies are to be involved in this field, since they must produce equipment that will fit in commercial systems. In addition, standards must be made for data transmission protocols.

Philips supports standards in most areas related to PAC systems. The only exception is in standards for data compression.

Device safety and liability

Hardware used in computer assisted medical imaging is generally controlled through national legislation on electricity (27). Companies have internal production standards, Good Manufacturing Practices (GMP), and often also meet national and international safety requirements. Equipment associated with ionizing radiation is often regulated as a special category. Legislation generally restricts and controls dosages of radiation given to patients and received by personnel working in imaging departments. Staff who use x-ray or nuclear imaging devices are required to have special training in the safety aspects of ionizing radiation and in the handling of equipment.

Some countries, for example the United States, regulate all devices for efficacy and safety before they can be marketed. The Netherlands, in contrast, has little regulatory control over devices on the market. However, the European Commission (EC) has issued guidelines for regulations for imaging equipment using ionizing radiation that must be followed by member countries. The Netherlands is now developing such regulations, and they may be expected to be implemented before 1990.

An important aspect of safety concerns equipment faults and malfunctions. These can lead to images of altered quality and can also increase exposure to ionizing radiation. Techniques for quality assurance of devices are therefore important.

Computers are generally unregulated, except for electrical safety. Likewise, computer software is generally not subject to regulation, although the U.S. Food and Drug Administration defines such software as a medical device.

Manufacturers attempt to assure adequate safety and performance for their products, in part for ethical reasons, in part to encourage sales and in part to avoid liability. In the United States, malpractice and product liability suits have made manufacturer's especially cautious. In other countries, similar legal provisions exist, but they are not used so actively by the public and the legal profession. Hospitals can also be liable for harm to patients, so have an incentive to be cautious in their approach to this field.

Section 5 – Conclusions

Computer assisted medical imaging is a rapidly growing aspect of health care. Its development has already begun to lead to profound changes in the traditional department of radiology. Even more dramatic changes seem likely in the future.

The most important implication of computer assisted imaging is that it uses digital data in producing images. Such data can be stored and manipulated by a computer and can be transmitted from place to place by data lines. The organization of the department of radiology is largely based on the fact of a physical film: an x-ray picture. This fact is now rapidly changing.

Computer assisted or digital imaging already makes up perhaps 20 percent of examinations in large hospitals, and perhaps 25 to 50 percent of images, indicating that more images per examination are taken with the new techniques (27, p. 50). At the same time, it accounts for only about 2 percent of the data in bits. As the percentage of digital examinations rises, and as the capability of storing, moving, and manipulating the data grows, a totally digitalized system (a PAC system) becomes more likely. At a minimum, it is clear that PAC systems will spread into use to handle the digital part of medical imaging. If conventional radiology becomes digital, this will also encourage PAC systems. It is also conceivable, even likely, that departments of medical imaging or radiology ultimately will become entirely digital.

This development raises several questions for policy makers:

1. When can PAC systems be expected to become mature?
2. Can health benefits be expected?
3. Is this development worthwhile for the system? Can efficiency benefits be anticipated? If PAC systems become mature, how much would they cost? Are the financial benefits large enough to allow the system to pay for itself?
4. If Dutch industry becomes more involved in computer assisted medical imaging, will that be of economic benefit to the country?
5. Can policy in the Netherlands encourage more rapid development of a fully integrated PACS? Should it?

This report has given some tentative answers to the these questions, in so far as seems possible at this moment. The policy conclusions that follow address needed actions in the Netherlands.

Conclusion 1. The government of the Netherlands and other policy making bodies should encourage the development of prototype PAC systems, integrated with digital imaging systems. Such encouragement should be closely coupled to an on-going evaluation plan.

The rapidity of developments described in this report is uncertain, but it does seem clear that computer assisted medical imaging and PAC systems will gradually become more important. Computer assisted medical imaging is already widely available and will certainly become more widely available. It seems likely that all radiology will be based on digital systems sometime in the future, perhaps before the year 2000.

PAC systems are somewhat more uncertain. Such systems seem possible technologically. Most observers predict that they will not be developed before 1995, but it is possible that technological developments will be more rapid. At the moment, such systems are quite expensive and their benefits are somewhat uncertain. As they mature technologically, benefits will become clearer and it will be possible to do careful cost analyses. Costs will almost certainly come down in time.

In any case, PAC systems will develop in other countries. The Netherlands is one country that has the capability to develop a PAC system that might be very competitive internationally.

So far in the Netherlands, the development of a prototype PAC system in Utrecht has involved a creative collaboration between a university hospital, the BAZIS organization, departments in several universities, industry, and government. Such collaboration should continue and grow, if PACS is to become successful soon in the Netherlands. An important aspect of this field at some point will be development and evaluation of a PACS for peripheral hospitals.

An important part of the developments so far has been a careful continuing evaluation (9). This is an innovative and praiseworthy development. It should be possible to devise an evaluation plan that would allow measurement of costs and benefits at each phase of installation or expansion (26).

One problem is the time it takes to develop needed technologies for a fully integrated PAC system. That problem will be solved during the next decade or so. Another problem in any country is the large amounts of capital investment needed. Using existing equipment, the cost to develop a system must be at least Dfl. 20 million. Ultimately, with equipment development, hundreds of millions of guilders will be required. Industry can make some of this investment, but government inevitably must make rather large investments if the effort is to succeed.

Different parts of the Dutch government could participate in such an effort. The Ministry of WVC has already funded the evaluation plan. The Ministry of Education and Science (O&W) could fund related research efforts, and also presently funds university hospitals, so could encourage or allow such developments through its funding. The Ministry of Economic Affairs (EZ) can encourage industry to become involved in new product development.

Conclusion 2. Industry needs to become actively involved in computer assisted medical imaging. Companies with specialized capabilities in computers, computer software, telecommunications, electronics, and so forth will find many opportunities for making components for PAC systems in the future. However, those opportunities can only exist if a sufficient degree of standardization has been reached.

It is often said in the Netherlands, by those who have some familiarity with local events, that PAC systems are developing, especially at Philips. It is said to be unnecessary to encourage Philips further. A role for other companies is not seen.

Such an attitude betrays a fundamental misunderstanding of the nature of the industrial role in computer assisted medical imaging and of the possible advantages for an expanded role. As pointed out in Section 2, perhaps no company has the ability to make all of the components necessary in computer assisted medical imaging. Subcontracting is common. Small specialized companies also have an important role.

From the standpoint of the Netherlands, such components will have to be purchased from outside if they are not made in the country. If they are made in the country, they will also be exported.

Conclusion 3. An ongoing commitment to research is needed, especially linking the stages of development of PACS to the value demonstrated for such systems. Evaluation research has already been mentioned. Research in electronics, computer programming, perception, simulation of systems, and data compression and transmission are also needed to reach an optimal PAC system.

The Netherlands has a relatively great capability for research in many areas related to PAC systems, especially through its technical universities. The potential of developing groups in which experts in medical sciences, health information systems, computers, and others work together collaboratively is relatively great. Such research needs to be encouraged as part of developing a fully integrated PAC system in the Netherlands.

Conclusion 4. Working with digital systems should become part of the training of all those who will use such systems before they become more widely available. This training is particularly important for radiologists.

It seems clear that digital imaging - and perhaps PACS itself - represents the future of radiology and medical imaging. No expert in medical imaging will be able to function effectively in the future without explicit training in these new systems.

In the long-run, such systems will certainly change roles of those involved in imaging. Medical imaging is already a multi-disciplinary activity because of the necessity for such skills as engineering and computer programming. One could foresee the possibility of significant changes in the functioning of different experts, such as radiologists.

Conclusion 5. Computer assisted medical imaging has considerable potential implications for health care delivery. These implications need to be monitored by policy makers for the purposes of strategic health planning.

It is not yet known when a fully integrated PACS will become available. Until one system is functioning, its implications will not be known. However, the long-term implications could be considerable, and are largely unforeseen. Policy makers should be prepared to intervene actively in this area if necessary. Possible interventions vary from active encouragement of systems that promise to increase efficiency to active discouragement of systems that have not been shown to have actual advantages.

Conclusion 6. International cooperation and information exchange is essential in the field of computer assisted medical imaging.

For a small country, effective involvement in computer assisted medical imaging will require international cooperation. Such cooperation should span all aspects of development and should focus on communication of information on research and development successes, availability of components, evaluation, and policy approaches to computer assisted imaging. A particularly critical issue in computer assisted imaging is standardization, and policy makers should encourage efforts to develop standards by any means possible. As in other areas of health care technology, the rapid developments in this field could leave behind a country that does not know international developments. The already existing Europacs organization, which originated from an initiative of the BAZIS group in Leiden, provides a forum for international cooperation. Its continuation should be assured financially. For the same reasons, funding should be available for researchers and developers in this field to visit other research centers and relevant conferences.

Computer assisted medical imaging is one of the most significant technologies to have developed during the last decades. Its full implications have only begun to be seen. In the future, dramatic and unforeseen consequences will follow from developments in the field of computer assisted imaging. Policy makers need to be aware of the potentials of this field and to monitor it closely. Both medical and financial benefits are possible, but these need to be demonstrated.

The benefits to Dutch society from computer assisted imaging could be great, both in the short- and the long-run.

Appendixes

APPENDIX A METHOD OF THE STUDY

The need for examining future health care technology was recognized by the Dutch Steering Committee on Future Health Scenarios (STG) in 1984. (The STG is an independent advisory group to the Dutch government set up in 1983 to carry out scenario studies as an aid to long-term health planning). The STG initiated the Project on Future Health Care Technology. The World Health Organization, European Office (WHO/EURO), agreed to support the project financially and logistically.

The project had two specific objectives:
1. To identify future technological developments in health care, with brief descriptions of potential technologies; and
2. To carry out prospective assessments of four high priority technologies or areas of technological development.

The project began in April 1985. A Commission on Future Health Care Technology made up of 10 members and 5 official observers was appointed to guide the project. Surveys of experts were carried out in the United States and Europe. The information from the surveys, supplemented by material from the scientific literature and from interviews, was the basis for the overall descriptions of health care technology. The assistance of these many individuals and groups is specifically acknowledged in appendixes to Volumes I and II of this report.

The project plan called for four technologies to be prospectively assessed. In September 1985, the Commission met and endorsed four cases:
1. implications of neurosciences;
2. biotechnology - probably examining both monoclonal antibodies and vaccines;
3. laser applications, especially in surgery and in the treatment of vascular disease, especially coronary artery disease; and
4. genetic testing

Later, with funding from the Ministry of Economic Affairs, medical imaging and home care technology were also developed as case studies.

A detailed description of methods for the entire project is presented in an appendix to Volume I of the report. An updated version may be found in Volume II. And each case study contains a methods description specific to that case.

Beginning in the fall of 1986, Dr. Taeke van Beekum of TNO began to work with the project one day a week on the home care and medical imaging cases. The staff for these two cases interviewed experts, made site visits, and collected materials during late 1986 and early 1987. In March 1987, a first complete draft of a report on computer-assisted medical image was completed. It was reviewed by Dr. de Valk and Dr. ter Haar Romeny and revised based on their comments. It was presented to a special working group session that discussed it at a special working group on 27 April 1987. Subsequent to that meeting, Mr. de Charro was given a small contract to revise the cost estimates in the report. These new materials were incorporated into the report in early May.

The final revisions were made, and the report was presented to the Commission. At a meeting on 18 May 1987, the Commission discussed the draft report and suggested some changes. It then approved the report with the understanding that it would be sent to the working group for one more review.

The report was revised after the Commission meeting and was sent to the working group for comments on 27 May 1987. Final comments were received by 10 June 1987. A few final changes in the report were made and it was submitted to the STG on 26 June 1987.

APPENDIX B GLOSSARY OF TERMS

Abscess: A circumscribed area of pus. A localized infection.

Algorithm: A procedure for solution of a mathematical problem in a finite number of steps. In practice, medical problems of diagnosis and therapy have been formulated into 'decision-trees.'
An algorithm is considered to be such a decision-tree or part of a decision-tree. Following a set of unambiguous questions and instructions that can be carried out one by one is expected to lead to a correct solution to a problem.

Analogue: Literally, something similar to something else. In computer assisted medical imaging, the term refers to keeping data obtained from an imaging procedure in picture form.

Angiography: A fluoroscopic examination for the imaging of blood vessels involving injection of a contrast medium into the veins.

Artificial intelligence: A field of research and development involving computers. The attempt is to develop programs that can reason and solve problems at a higher level than is now possible.

Biopsy: Examination of tissues, normal or abnormal, excised from the living body.

Byte: A group of digits often shorter than a word that a computer processes as a unit.

Central nervous system: The brain and spinal cord. The nerves and ganglia outside of the central nervous system constitute the peripheral nervous system.

Clinical trial: An experiment carried out for the purpose of evaluating the efficacy and safety of a health care technology. The nature of the control group is a critical issue in a clinical trial. See **Control group, Randomized clinical trial.**

Computer assisted medical imaging: The field of producing pictures of the inside of the living human body using techniques involving computers. Traditionally, the field was called 'radiology' to refer to the usual modality, x-rays. With the advent of modern technologies such as CT scanning and NMR scanning, the term 'imaging' is more often used.

Computed tomography (CT) scanner: A diagnostic device that combines X-ray equipment with a computer and a display monitor to produce images of cross-sections of the body. Also called 'computerized axial tomography (CAT) scanner.'

Control group: In a randomized clinical trial, the group receiving no treatment or some treatment with which the group receiving experimental treatment is compared. The control treatment is generally a standard treatment, a placebo, or no treatment. Compare **Experimental group**.

Controlled clinical trial: See **Clinical trial**.

Cost-effectiveness analysis (CEA): An analytical technique that compares the costs of a project or of alternative projects to the resultant benefits, with costs and benefits/effectiveness expressed by different measures. Costs are usually expressed in financial terms, but benefits/effectiveness are ordinarily expressed in terms such as 'lives saved,' 'disability avoided,' 'quality-adjusted life years saved,' or any other relevant objectives.

CT scanner: See **Computed tomography scanner**.

Data compression: Electronic compression of the data involved in a computer assisted medical image. Data compression is an essential part of PACS, since the large amounts of data produced in a fully digitized system would be difficult to transmit over distances.

Digital (digitalization or digitization): A term that refers to data in numeric form. Digital data is manipulable by computer, so its use is growing rapidly in health care. One rapidly growing application is in medical imaging, where analogue data (similar to the structure examined, as with a chest x-ray) is converted to digital form and stored and manipulated by a computer.

Digital substraction angiography: A type of imaging of the blood vessels based on the use of digital images. Contrast material is injected into the veins and images before and during the passage of the contrast material are compared by subtracting one from the other. The result is that image areas where no changes occurred are wiped out and only the contrast bearing vessels become clearly visible. Thus, lesions within the vessels can be imaged clearly.

Effectiveness: Same as efficacy (see below) except that it refers to '...average or actual conditions of use.'

Efficacy: The probability of benefit to individuals in a defined population from a medical technology applied for a given medical problem under ideal conditions of use.

Ergonomics: The study of the work performed by a muscle or group of muscles. Ergonomics involves studying the posture of the body and effort expended by muscles to assure that the design of equipment is acceptable for human functioning.

Experimental group: In a randomized clinical trial, the group receiving the treatment being evaluated for safety and efficacy. The experimental treatment may be a new technology, an existing technology applied to a new problem, or an accepted treatment about whose safety or efficacy there is doubt. Compare **Control group**.

Expert system: A computer program in which the knowledge of experts is stored in such a way that it can be retrieved for problem-solving. Expert systems are available to aid both medical diagnosis and medical treatment.

False negative: A negative test result in an individual who actually **does have** the disease or characteristic being tested for. The person is incorrectly diagnosed as not having a particular disease or characteristic.

False positive: A positive test result in an individual who does **not** have the disease or characteristic being tested for. I.e., the individual is incorrectly diagnosed as having a particular disease or characteristic.

Fluorescent: Having the property of emitting electromagnetic radiation, usually visible light, when exposed to radiation from another source.

Fluoroscopy: Imaging of the body with x-ray. The image is acquired using an image intensifier that displays the image on a screen. Dynamic events, such as the beating of the heart, can be seen using this technique. Cine or video cameras can be connected to the output screen to record the output for later analysis.

Gamma radiation: A form of ionizing radiation similar to x-rays.

Gray scale: A measure of the functional value of a pixel. Radiographic image gray scale values correspond to some physical properties of the structures in the objected imaged. In an image obtained by digitizing an x-ray film, for example, the gray scale value of a pixel corresponds to the optical density of that specific area of the film.

Health care technology: The drugs, devices, and medical and surgical procedures used in medical care, and the organizational and support systems within which such care is provided.

Hospital information system: A computer-based record-keeping system used in hospitals. Hospitals found increasing difficulties coordinating and communicating the massive quantities of data involved in hospital care, which led to systems based on computers. The first systems incorporated only administrative and financial data, but increasingly, clinical data is being included in such systems.

Image intensifier: A device that enhances the brightness of an image without increasing radiation dose.

Image processing: Manipulation of the image in computer assisted medical imaging. Since the image is based on numerical data, it can be manipulated by special computer programs.

Imaging: See **Medical imaging.**

Innovation: A new device, product, or process introduced to practice for the first time. Innovations are valued for their capacity to improve the quality or decrease the costs of a given process or product. Also, something perceived to be new. In addition, innovation is widely used to refer to the process by which technological change occurs.

Ionizing radiation: A form of radiant energy within the electromagnetic spectrum that has the capability of penetrating solid objects and altering the electrical charge of their atoms. X-rays and gamma rays are examples of ionizing radiation. Ionizing radiation is associated with certain dangers, including the possibility of inducing cancer.

Juke box: A device that holds multiple disks and can select the appropriate one on command. A juke box is an essential part of the archiving system of a PACS based on optical discs.

Laser: A light device that produces a highly focussed, high power source of energy that can be directed at a specific target point. Lasers are being applied to many areas of medicine, including surgery.

Lesion: Structural change in a tissue or organ.

Magnetic resonance imaging: See **Nuclear magnetic resonance**.

Medical imaging: The field of producing pictures of the inside of the living human body. Traditionally, the field was called 'radiology' to refer to the usual modality, X-rays. With the advent of modern technologies such as CT scanning and NMR scanning, this term is being used more and more frequently. See **Computed tomography scanning**, **Nuclear magnetic resonance**, **Ultrasound**, and **Positron emission tomography**.

Mutagenic: Causing mutations. Associated with changes in the structure of DNA, the genetic material of the cell.

Noninvasive technique: A diagnostic method that does not involve the penetration (by surgery or hypodermic needle) of the skin.

Nuclear magnetic resonance: A phenomenon in which atoms can be induced, by use of a magnetic field, to emit energy. The energy that is emitted can be used to produce images of structures inside the living body for diagnostic purposes.

Nuclear magnetic resonance spectroscopy: Energy produced by nuclear magnetic resonance can also be used to analyze the chemical composition of, and thus the metabolic processes in, tissues. This is now being used experimentally, and is expected to have important medical applications.

Nuclear medicine: An imaging technique in which radioactive 'tracers' are injected into the body. The tracer distributes itself in the body, and the radioactivity emitted is used to produce medical images.

PACS: See **Picture Archiving and Communication System.**

Picture Archiving and Communication System (PACS): A system of image storage, transmission and display based on digital imaging.

Pixel: Picture element. The term is used to express the number of picture elements in an image.

Positron-emission tomography (PET): A noninvasive scanning technique that images the uptake of radioactively labeled substances emitting subatomic particles (positrons). PET scans provide a dynamic picture of an organ's metabolic activity, as opposed to computed tomography (CT) scans, which yield a static anatomical view of the parts being examined.

Prospective assessment: Assessment of a technology before it has been developed. Later in the life-cycle of the technology, data can be collected to make these assessments more realistic. A prospective assessment is, by definition, somewhat speculative. Nonetheless, it may be helpful for planning.

Radiation: A form of energy within the electromagnetic spectrum. See also **Ionizing radiation.**

Radioactive: Having radioactivity.

Radioactive isotope: A term that refers to a form of an element that is chemically identical to other forms of the element but that has a slightly different atomic weight and that is unstable. Such forms of the element have a tendency to move to lower energy states, and when they do, they emit radiation.

Radioactivity: The property of emitting rays or particles (e.g., gamma rays, alpha particles, beta particles) of matter which can pass through various substances opaque of light rays and which can cause chemical and electrical effects.

Radiolabelling: Refers to the attachment of a radioactive substance to another substance for the purpose of following its distribution or measuring its concentration in the body.

Radiologist: The medical specialist who supervises medical imaging procedures and interprets the images for diagnostic purposes.

Radionuclide: A radioactive substance (or tracer) produced for the purpose of a nuclear medicine diagnostic procedure. See **Nuclear medicine**.

Radiopharmaceutical: A drug that has been labelled with a radioactive substance. See **Radiolabelling**.

Radiotherapy: Treatment by radioactivity or ionizing radiation (e.g., x-rays), most commonly used in cancer therapy.

Randomized clinical trial (RCT): An experiment designed to test the safety and efficacy of a medical technology in which people are randomly allocated to experimental or control groups, and outcomes are compared.

Resolution: See **Spatial resolution**.

Risk: A measure of the probability of an adverse or untoward outcome and the severity of the resultant harm to health of individuals in a defined population and associated with the use of a medical technology applied for a given medical problem under specified conditions of use.

Safety: A judgment of the acceptability of risk in a specified situation. See also **Risk**.

Scenario: An account of the present situation of a society or a part thereof, of possible and desirable alternative future situations of that society, and of alternative sequences of events that from present circumstances could lead to such futures.

Screening: An attempt to detect high risk individuals or those with disorders that have not yet caused symptoms. Screening is followed by specific diagnostic procedures when positive. It is done for the purpose of intervention, i.e., to cure the disease or prevent problems associated with it.

Sensitivity: The true positive ratio. In referring to a diagnostic test, it is the extent to which abnormals are correctly classified (positive test results divided by the number of patients who actually have the disease).

Somatic: A term used to refer to body tissues apart from reproductive (germinal) tissues.

Spatial resolution: The extent to which two adjacent structures can be distinguished, especially in a medical image.

Specificity: The true negative ratio. In referring to a diagnostic test, it is the extent to which normals are correctly classified (negative test results divided by the number of patients that actually have the disease). Compare **sensitivity**.

Technology: The application of organized knowledge to practical ends.

Technology assessment: In general, a comprehensive form of policy research that examines the technical, economic, and social consequences of technological applications. It is especially concerned with unintended, indirect, or delayed social impacts. In health policy, however, the term more often is used to mean any form of policy analysis concerned with health care technology, especially the evaluation of efficacy and safety.

Technology diffusion: The diffusion or spread of a medical technology into the health care system. It is generally thought to involve two phases: the initial phase in which decisions are made to adopt or reject the technology, and a subsequent phase in which decisions are made to use the technology.

Telecommunications: Communication at a distance through various means, including telegraph, telephone wire, or satellite. At present, a computer is often part of a communication system.

Telediagnostics: Diagnosis at a distance, using telecommunications.

Telemetry: The science or process of transmitting quantitative measurements (such as pressure, speed, or temperature) by radio to a distant site where the measurements are recorded.

Teleradiology: The electronic transmission of medical images over a distance, between clinics, other remote facilities, or other units in a hospital and a department of radiology.

Tomographic scan: The image of an individual slice or plane, usually through the body.

Transducer: A device actuated by power from one system that supplies power, usually in another form, to a second system. In ultrasound imaging, the transducer converts electrical energy to high frequency sound waves.

Ultrasound: High frequency sound waves that can be focussed and used to picture tissues, organs, structures, or tumors within the body. Ultrasound is particularly useful for in utero examination of the fetus and placenta. It is also increasingly used in the diagnosis of heart diseases and other vascular diseases.

X-ray: A form of high energy electromagnetic energy used to produce images of the human body. See also **Ionizing radiation**.

APPENDIX C REFERENCES

1. Abrams H, McNeil B. Medical implications of computed tomography ("CT scanning"). New England Journal of Medicine 1978; 298: 255-261, 310-318.

2. van Aken IW, Reijns GL, de Valk JPJ, Nijhof JAM. Compressed medical images and enhanced fault detection within an ACR-NEMA compatible picture archiving and communications system. In: Schneider RH, Dwyer SJ eds. Proceedings Medical Imaging Conference. The International Society for Optical Engineering (SPIE) 1987; 767: Paper number 34.

3. Ambrose J, Gooding MR. E.M.I. scan in the management of head injuries. Lancet 1976; 1: 847-849.

4. Anbar M, Schersten T. Computer assisted clinical decisions: present scope, limitations and future. International Journal of Technology Assessment in Health Care 1986; 2: 168-176.

5. Bailey R. Patient exposure requirements for high resolution in digital radiographic systems. American Journal of Radiology 1984; 142: 603-608.

6. Bakker AR, Didden H, de Valk JPJ, Bijl K. Traffic load on the image storage component in a PACS. In: Schneider RH, Dwyer SJ eds. Proceedings Medical Imaging Conference. The International Society for Optical Engineering (SPIE) 1987; 767: Paper number 94.

7. Banta HD. The diffusion of the computed tomography (CT) scanner in the United States. International Journal of Health Services 1980; 10: 251-269.

8. Banta HD. Embracing or rejecting innovations: clinical diffusion of health care technology. In: Reiser SJ, Anbar M, eds. The machine at the bedside. London: Cambridge University Press, 1984: 65-92.

9. Banta HD, Behney CJ. Policy formulation and technology assessment. Milbank Memorial Fund Quarterly/Health and Society 1981; 59: 445-479.

10. Banta HD, Behney CJ, Willems JS. Toward rational technology in medicine. New York: Springer Publishing Company, 1981.

11. Banta HD, McNeil BJ. Evaluation of the CAT scanner and other diagnostic technologies. Health Care Management Review 1978; 3: 7-19.

12. Bautz W, Kolbe J. Ist ein PACS fur eine grosse radiologische Abteilung realisierbar? Uberlegungen anhand des Bilddatenaufkommens des medizinischen Strahleninstituts der Universitat Tubingen im Jahr 1983. Digitale Bilddiagnose 1986; 6: 43-48.

13. van Bemmel JH. Man and computer in the hospital of tomorrow. Amsterdam: Department of Medical Informatics, Free University of Amsterdam, 1985.

14. Bijl K, Koens ML, Bakker AR, de Valk JPJ. Medical PACS and HIS: integration needed! In: Schneider RH, Dwyer SJ eds. Proceedings Medical Imaging Conference. The International Society for Optical Engineering (SPIE) 1987; 767: Paper number 89.

15. Bloom KJ, Weinstein RS. Expert systems: robot physicians of the future? Human Pathology 1985; 16: 1082-1084.

16. Brauer GW. The fully-computerized medical imaging department in a community hospital: a technology assessment. Presented at the Third Annual Meeting, International Society of Technology Assessment in Health Care, Rotterdam, May 21-22, 1987.

17. van den Brink JV. What radiologists say about PACS. American Journal of Radiology 1986; 146:419-420.

18. Burke MW, Ackerman LV. Cooperation between a radiology computer consortium and a computer manufacturer in the development of a radiology information system. Henry Ford Hospital Medical Journal 1984; 32: 188-190.

19. Capp MP, Roehrig H, Seeley GW, Fisher HD, Ovitt TW. The digital radiology department of the future. Radiological Clinics of North America 1985; 23: 349-355.

20. Cocklin M, Gourlay A, Jackson P, Kaye G, Miessler M, Kerr I, Lams P. An image processing system for digital chest x-ray images. Computer Programs in Biomedicine 1984; 19: 3-11.

21. Cox GC, Templeton AW, Dwyer SJ. Digital image management: networking, display, and archiving. Use of Computers in Radiology 1986; 24: 37-54.

22. Dahlin H, Hamren M. CART - computer aided radio therapy. Presentation of an integrated information system in radiotherapy. Report from the NORDFORSK Project, Uppsala, 1984.

23. Drew PG. Picture archiving and communication systems. Chicago: American Hospital Association, 1985.

24. Drew PG. Picture archiving and communication systems. Hospitals 1985; 4: 78,79,82,86.

25. Drew PG. Putting the squeeze on images through data compression. Diagnostic Imaging 1986; 8: 142-143.

26. Drummond M, Cockshott P, Haynes B, Walter S. Guidelines for the evaluation of digital diagnostic imaging equipment or units. Report submitted to Health and Welfare Canada, 24 March 1983.

27. Economic Commission for Europe, United Nations. Working Party on Engineering Industries and Automation. Digital imaging in health care. New York, 1987. ISBN 92-1-116 380-3.

28. ECRI. Digital imaging storage and retrieval in the 1980s: a preliminary assessment. Journal of Health Care Technology 1984; 1: 13-38.

29. ECRI. Image transmission and data compression, two key elements of an electronic imaging department. Health Care Technology 1986; 3: 83-93.

30. ECRI. X-ray image digitizing systems. Issues in Health Care Technology. New Technology Briefs/5.D.4, 1984.

31. Erdman WA, Maguire GQ, Noz ME et al. PACS: modus operandi for filmless nuclear medicine department. Administrative Radiology 1986; 5: 34-36, 38.

32. A European Workshop Sponsored by the EEC. Methodology of Positron Emission Tomography. London, March 1984.

33. Fieschi M, Joubert M. Some reflections of the evaluation of expert systems in medicine. Meth. Inform. Med. 1986; 25: 15-21.

34. Fineberg H, Bauman R, Sosman. Computerized cranial tomography: effect on diagnostic and therapeutic plans. Journal of the American Medical Association 1977; 238: 224-227.

35. Gezondheidsraad. NMR - vorming en opleiding. The Hague, The Netherlands. 13 July 1985.

36. Gezondheidsraad. Opleiding ultra-geluid. The Hague, The Netherlands. 29 November 1985.

37. Gray JE, Karsell PR, Becker GP, Gehring DG. Total digital radiology: is it feasible? or desirable? American Journal of Radiology 1984; 143: 1345-1349.

38. Greinacher CFC. Siemens & PACS. EuroPACS Newsletter, Leiden, Volume 2, Number 1, September 1986: 27-31.

39. Greinacher CFC, Muller K, Fuchs D. Digitale Bildinformationssysteme in der Radiologie - Stand und Entwicklungstendenzen. Digitale Bilddiagnose 1984; 4: 87-104.

40. ter Haar Romeny BM, de Graaff CN, van Waes PFGM, van Rijk PP, Helder JC, de Valk JPJ. Beeld opslag en communicatie systemen voor ziekenhuizen. Klinische Fysica 1986; Number 1: 1-11.

41. Hindel R. Review of optical storage technology for archiving digital medical images. Radiology 1986; 161: 257-262.

42. Hintze VA, Jotten G. Digitale Radiographie. Fortschritt in Rontgenstralung 186; 145: 91-97.

43. Hoehne KH. Pictorial information systems in medicine. Berlin: Springer-Verlag, 1984.

44. Huang HK. Biomedical image processing. CRC Critical Reviews in Biomedical Engineering 1981; 5: 185-271.

45. Huang HK. Elements of digital radiology. New York: Prentice-Hall, 1986.

46. Jain AK. Image data compression: a review. Proceedings of the IEEE 1981; 69: 349-389.

47. James AE, Carroll F, Pickens DR, Chapman JC, Robinson RR, Pendergrass HP, Zaner R. Medical image management. Radiology 1986; 160: 411-416.

48. Kalisman M, Kalisman A. Data storage and retrieval. Computers in Plastic Surgery 1986; 13: 529-543.

49. Kastan DJ, Ackerman LV, Feczko PJ, Beute GH. Digital radiography: a review. Henry Ford Hospital Medical Journal 1985; 33: 88-94.

50. Kulikowski CA. Expert medical consultation systems. Journal of Medical Systems 1983; 7: 229-234.

51. Lamm IL, Dahlin H, Moller T. CART - A Nordic challenge in medical computing. Computers in Radiotherapy and Oncology; March 1984: 81-86.

52. McGrohan L, Patterson JF, Gagne RM, Goldstein HA. Average radiation doses in a standard head examination for 250 CT systems. Radiology 1987; 163: 263-268.

53. Massar ADA, de Valk JPJ, Reijns GL, Bakker AR. Simulation of an image network in a medical image information system. In: Sutens P, Young IT eds. The International Society for Optical Engineering (SPIE) 1985; 593: 123-131.

54. Menkin M, DeFriese GH, Oliver TR, Litt I. The cost effectiveness of digital subtraction angiography in the diagnosis of cerebrovascular disease. Office of Technology Assessment. Health Technology Case Study 34. Washington DC: US Government Printing Office, 1985.

55. Moores BM. The third symposium on PACS and PHD and fifth symposium on medical imaging technology, Japan. EuroPACS Newsletter, Leiden, Volume 2, Number 1, September 1986: 33-35.

56. Noz ME, Erdman WA, Maguire GQ. Local area networks in an imaging environment. CRC Critical Reviews in Medical Information 1986; 1: 81-133.

57. Noz ME, Maguire GQ, Horii SC, Zeleznik MP, Schimpf JH, Baxter BS. A distribution system for digital images from diverse image sources. Incorporating a local area network in an imaging environment. Journal of Medical Systems 1983; 7: 349-361.

58. Noz ME, Erdman WA, Maguire GQ, Stahl TJ, Tokarz RJ, Menken KL, Salviani JA. Modus operandi for a picture archiving and communication system. Radiology 1984; 152: 221-223.

59. Office of Technology Assessment. Nuclear magnetic resonance imaging technology, a clinical, industrial, and policy analysis. Health Technology Case Study 27. Washington DC: US Government Printing Office, 1984.

60. Office of Technology Assessment. Policy implications of the computed tomography (CT) scanner. Washington DC: US Government Printing Office, 1978.

61. Office of Technology Assessment. Policy implications of the computed tomography (CT) scanner: an update. Washington DC: US Government Printing Office, 1981.

62. Rabbani M, Ray LA, Sullivan JR. Adaptive predictive coding with applications to radiographs. Medical Instrumentation 1986; 20: 182-191.

63. Reggia JA. Medical decision support systems: from theory to practice. Medical Informatics 1984; 9: 223-230.

64. Reiser SJ. Medicine and the reign of technology. London: Cambridge University Press, 1978.

65. Riederer SJ. Digital radiography. CRC Critical Reviews in Biomedical Engineering 1985; 12: 163-200.

66. Seeley GW, Ovitt T, Capp MP. The total digital radiology department: an alternative view (editorial). American Journal of Radiology 1985; 144: 421-422.

67. Seeley GW, Newell JD. The use of psychophysical principles in the design of a total digital radiology department. Radiologic Clinics of North America 1985; 23: 341-348.

68. Stason WB, Fortess E. Case study #13: Cardiac radionuclide imaging and cost effectiveness. The implications of cost-effectiveness analysis of medical technology. Washington DC: US Government Printing Office, 1982.

69. Stevens R. American medicine and the public interest. New Haven: Yale University Press, 1971.

70. Stevens R. Medical practice in modern England. New Haven: Yale University Press, 1966.

71. Ter-Pogossian MM et al. Positron-Emission Tomography. Scientific American 1980; 243: 170-186.

72. de Valk JPJ, Bakker AR, Bijl D, Heijser W, Boekee DE. PACS reviewed: possible and coming soon? EuroPACS Newsletter, Leiden, Volume 2, Number 1, September 1986: 36-39.

73. de Valk JPJ, Bakker AR, Bijl D, Heijser W, Boekee DE. PACS reviewed: possible and coming soon? Journal of Medical Imaging 1987; 2: 77-84.

74. de Valk JPJ, ter Haar Romeny BM, Reichwein ABPJ. Beeldopslag en communicatie systemen voor ziekenhuizen (PACS), een overzicht. Techniek in de Gezondheidszorg 1986; 11: 9-13.

75. de Valk JPJ, Kroon HMJA, Boekee DE, Reijns GL, van Erning LJTO, Seeley GW, Reemer R, Tor RCG, Bakker AR. The set up of a diagnostic image quality evaluation chain. In: Schneider RH, Dwyer SJ eds. Proceedings Medical Imaging Conference. The International Society for Optical Engineering (SPIE) 1987; 767: Paper number 90.

76. de Valk JPJ, van Rijnsoever RC, Bakker AR. Simulation of a feasible medical image storage hierarchy within the Dutch IMAGIS project. In: Sprague RA, Bell AE, de Haan MR, Jamberdino AA eds. Proceedings Third International Conference on Optical Mass Data Storage. SPIE 1985; 529: 240-244.

77. Wilson P. Digital imaging: an introduction. Radiography 1984; 50: 44-49.

78. Witte VC, Hoehne KH, Boecker F, Riemer M, Bucheler E. Ansendungsmoglichkeiten digitaler Methoden in der Rontgendiagnostik. Fortschr. Rontgenstr. 1985; 142: 600-610.

79. Yu VL. Conceptual obstacles in computerized medical diagnosis. Journal of Medicine and Philosophy 1983; 8: 67-75.

APPENDIX D ACKNOWLEDGEMENTS

Working Group on Computer Assisted Medical Imaging

Prof.dr. L.H.J.F. Beckmann
BV Optische Industrie
'De Oude Delft'

Dr. D.E. Boekee
Faculteit der Electrotechniek
Technical University of Delft

F.T.M. de Charro
Faculteit Rechtsgeleerdheid
Erasmus Universiteit

Ir. C. Kramer
Medical Systems
Philips Nederland

Ir. B.M. Ter Haar-Romeny
Centrale Rontgen
Academisch Ziekenhuis Utrecht

Dr. J.P.J. de Valk
BAZIS Project
Academisch Ziekenhuis Leiden

Ir. P.A. Vis (observer)
Ministerie van Economische Zaken

Prof. A.E. van Voorthuisen
Faculteit der Geneeskunde
Rijksuniversiteit Utrecht

Dr.P.F.G.M. van Waes
Faculteit der Geneeskunde
Rijksuniversiteit Utrecht

Dr.ir. P. Zuidema
Sector Informatica en Automatisering
Ministerie van WVC

Contractors

F.T.M. de Charro assisted with the cost estimates in Section 3.

The total output of the project is as follows:

Volume 1	General Considerations and Policy Conclusions
Volume 2	Future Technological Changes
Volume 3	Developments in the Regeneration, Repair and Reorganization of Nervous Tissue
Volume 4	Health Care Applications of Lasers: The Future Treatment of Coronary Artery Disease
Volume 5	Developments in Genetic Testing
Volume 6	Applications of the New Biotechnology: The Case of Vaccines
Volume 7	Computer-Assisted Medical Imaging
Volume 8	Potentials for Home Care Technology

FSC
www.fsc.org
MIX
Papier | Fördert gute Waldnutzung
FSC® C083411

Kolibri 360 GmbH
Ferdinand-Jühlke-Straße 7
99095 Erfurt, Deutschland
produktsicherheit@kolibri360.de